The
Nevertheless
Principle

Other books by Marion Bond West

Out of My Bondage
No Turning Back
Two of Everything But Me
Learning to Lean

Marion Bond West

The Nevertheless Principle

Published by

chosen books

FLEMING H. REVELL COMPANY
OLD TAPPAN, NEW JERSEY

The Scripture reference used is the King James Version, unless otherwise noted.
The material in chapter 4 appeared in a longer version as "The Loving Arms of God" in
Guideposts magazine, November 1983, for which grateful acknowledgment is made.

Library of Congress Cataloging-in-Publication Data

West, Marion B.
    The nevertheless principle.

    "Chosen books."
    1. West, Jerry M. (Jerry Michael), 1935-1983.
2. West, Marion B. 3. Christian life—1960-
4. Christian biography—United States. 5. Brain—Cancer—Patients
—United States—Biography. I. Title.
BR1725.W416W47   1986   280'.4 [B]   86-10188
ISBN 0-8007-9057-X

For Jerry . . .
just as I promised
July 1983

Table of Contents

Preface

For almost as long as I can remember, I have been plagued with thoughts that begin with *What if . . .* ? Usually such thought attacks come in the middle of the night, although they can sneak up in the daytime, too.

"What if Jennifer's had a wreck . . . ?"

"What if the little lump is more than just a lump . . . ?"

"What if my husband doesn't love me anymore . . . ?"

"What if . . . ?"

"What if . . . ?"

Some of the what-ifs I can't even make myself put on paper. Any what-if nourished with proper thought and imagination can grow to hideous proportions.

In October 1982, a what-if in my life presented itself with terrifying probability. My husband and I were about to celebrate our twenty-fifth wedding anniversary. All the years had not been good ones. We had had problems, the oldest being a lack of communication.

"Talk to me," I had begged Jerry for years. Now we were about to face a situation that made our previous problems small by comparison. The doctor, eager to get it over with, said, "Your husband came through the surgery fine, but I could remove only part of a malignant brain tumor. He has a few months at most."

The doctor talked on and on, saying all that doctors are required to say in such situations, but his words made no sense. Jerry was 47 years old; he had never been sick a day in his life. He couldn't die! If he did, how could I go on living?

It was seven long months before the answer came. It was only one word. But there was deep theology and many Scriptures to back it up. From that single word came courage and finally joy. Perhaps life did still hold meaning. Maybe I could laugh again. With that word a great change began inside me. I knew what I looked like on the inside—a city after a hydrogen bomb hit, everything dead and gray and covered in ashes. Nothing moved. No life was ever expected again. And then in that hopeless desolation on May 11, 1983, a small green shoot emerged. It was new and tender and only one word tall.

Nevertheless.

Swiftly it took root in my mind until a sentence appeared: *God is not a God of what-if; He is the God of nevertheless.* It was a powerful little sentence.

Never the less.

Nevertheless with God, no matter what, always the most. No matter what has happened! I began to think, dream, breathe *nevertheless.* Obsessed with the word, I started to research it in the concordance, finding it used in the Bible more than ninety times, almost always with tremendous power:

". . . Then they were very wroth, And conspired all of them together to come and to fight against Jerusalem. . . . Nevertheless we made our prayer unto our God" (Nehemiah 4:7–9).

"For I said in my haste, I am cut off from before thine eyes: nevertheless thou heardest the voice of my supplications when I cried unto thee" (Psalm 31:22).

"So foolish was I, and ignorant: I was as a beast before thee. Nevertheless I am continually with thee" (Psalm 73:22–23).

"Nevertheless my loving-kindness will I not utterly take from him, nor suffer my faithfulness to fail" (Psalm 89:33).

Simon's response when Jesus instructs him to launch out into the deep: "Master, we have toiled all the night, and have taken nothing: nevertheless at thy word I will let down the net'' (Luke 5:5).

Jesus' response when the Pharisees warn Him that Herod is determined to kill Him: "Nevertheless I must walk to-day and to-morrow . . .'' (Luke 13:32).

When Jesus gathers His disciples in the Upper Room: "Nevertheless I tell you the truth; It is expedient for you that I go away: for if I go not away, the Comforter will not come unto you" (John 16:7).

When Jesus cries out in anguish to his Father: ". . . Take away this cup from me: nevertheless, not what I will, but what thou wilt" (Mark 14:36).

After Jesus' resurrection: ". . . We were troubled on every side; without were fightings, within were fears. Nevertheless God, that comforteth those that are cast down, comforted us . . ." (2 Corinthians 7:5–6).

"For the which cause I also suffer these things: nevertheless I am not ashamed . . ." (2 Timothy 1:12).

"I am crucified with Christ: nevertheless I live . . . by the faith of the Son of God, who loved me, and gave himself for me" (Galatians 2:20).

So my Bible search bore out what I suspected. *Nevertheless* was no ordinary lifestyle. It was a supernatural way to live, no matter what life dished out—a power and a dimension that seemed to be reserved mainly for the desperate.

I qualified!

Further, meditating on these Scriptures, I saw that thoughts beginning with what-if *never* came from God, but from the enemy, the fear monster. Was it possible that he could be destroyed by one powerful, God-given word turned into a lifestyle?

From the almost unbelievable change in my life since I discovered that God is not a God of what-if but the God of nevertheless, I knew someone must write this book. I confess openly that I don't know how. I feel inadequate and I probably am. It is a tremendous undertaking, 'way too big for me. That I have written four other books doesn't seem to help a bit. I have never felt such a mixture of excitement and helplessness.

Nevertheless, I have begun.

Marion Bond West
Lilburn, Georgia

Foreword

I let out a groan as I drew the manuscript from its wrapping and skimmed the opening chapter. (Such careful wrapping! Three layers of brown paper around a masking-taped box, more protective sheets inside.) One more account by a courageous widow. . . . I turned the typed pages faster. It was all there: details of a husband's final days, the ensuing battle with grief.

These submissions come over every editor's desk, perhaps more often than any other kind of story. The problem is not that they are poorly written—most are beautifully expressed. Or unimportant—they deal with one of the most profound of all human experiences. It is simply that they are very, very familiar: as familiar as death, and the love that wants to remember.

And so the editor glances through them with regret, moved by their earnestness, groping for words with which to cushion the letter of rejection. "Your husband was clearly a wonderful person, but unfortunately we have similar book proposals which. . . ."

The letter wrote itself in my head as I scanned *The Nevertheless Principle*. It was late, bedtime. If the decision were less routine I would never have started a manuscript at 11:00 at night. But after all, a widow eulogizing a husband's memory. . . .

Three hours later, with a very stiff back, I laid down one of the most remarkable narratives I had ever read. Death of a husband?

Adjustment to windowhood? These were the specific setting for the story, but they were not the subject matter.

The subject was fear. Not fear of anything in particular, but fearfulness itself. That nagging, ever-shifting, joy-robbing apprehensiveness that haunts so many of us all our lives. It had me. It had many people I knew. And it had Marion Bond West, author of the manuscript in front of me.

For Marion, fear took the form of "what-if?" "What if my husband loses his job?" "What if my daughter has an accident?"

A committed Christian, Marion didn't have much trouble recognizing the big sins, the big temptations. Those insinuating little what-ifs, however, slipped behind her defenses, whispering to her at night, invading her very prayer times, stealing her peace.

Then, into Marion's life came a what-if of terrifying probability. An inoperable brain tumor was diagnosed in her athletic 47-year-old husband. *What if* Jerry died? *What if* he suffered terribly? *What if* she had to raise the children alone?

Faced with the worst thing she could imagine, this woman so given to fearful imaginings fell apart as promptly and thoroughly as she knew she would. How her life came together again—while every outer circumstance grew worse—is a story of such tremendous practical application, based on such solid biblical authority, that I put down the final page at two in the morning with a sense of strange excitement.

Too stimulated to go to bed, I went into the kitchen and put on a pot of coffee. A key of tremendous importance had just been placed in my hands, and I wanted to think about it. I was sure it was a key not only to the great soul-searing crises, like Marion's, but to the small everyday ones, too. *The Nevertheless Principle*, I suspected, would go to work in my life the very next day.

Sooner. It was late, as I say, and I had a busy day coming up. *What if* I'm too tired to go to work? The question had barely surfaced when I began to laugh. *"What-if,"* I told that little anxiety, "there's a principle I'd like you to know about."

Elizabeth Sherrill
Chosen Books

Acknowledgments

A fter three rewrites, *The Nevertheless Principle* had become like an emotional hot potato. I knew I had to release it and that someone very special was needed to do the laborious task of editing. I had no idea who that someone would be.

As I put the carefully wrapped and much-prayed-over manuscript in the mail, I related to Moses' mother as she placed her beloved baby into a basket and relinquished him. I so wanted to hold onto the manuscript, but that was impossible.

Surely God had Elizabeth Sherrill, my own Miriam, at the edge of the river waiting quietly and watching for a bundle that had been almost impossible to release. Hudson Taylor was right! God reserves the very best for those who leave the choice to Him.

For professional reasons, all doctors' names have been changed. I have only admiration and gratitude for their care and concern for Jerry and me. He received excellent treatment and we grew to love all fifteen of the doctors we came in contact with. My deep gratitude goes out also to DeKalb General Hospital, Decatur, Georgia, and everyone there with whom we came in contact.

Introduction

T*he Nevertheless Principle* traces the journey from despair and hopelessness to peace and joy. To reach Nevertheless Living, one must travel the dreaded road of fear and deep depression. There is no other route and no shortcut. The secret of arriving at the much-desired goal is to keep moving along when there no longer seems to be any purpose in moving. The rewards of Nevertheless Living are so intense that it is worth whatever the cost.

For, strangely, it is people who have been terribly hurt, even devastated, who seem to enter most readily into Nevertheless Living—not those who are already experiencing "normal" peace, love and contentment. It is reserved for those who are more than conquerors through God's marvelous grace.

One cannot arrive at Nevertheless Living by being smart or strong or determined, by fighting or by willpower. The paradox is that you get there by simply giving up and entering a stage of trust that staggers the imagination.

Once you enter Nevertheless Living, you know it. You are in another dimension, as surely as men who travel in space find themselves weightless. For you, life has started all over. You have become another person in the same body. It's fun getting to know yourself. You are fear-free. The worst thing that could possibly happen has happened, and you are flooded with joy and a strange sense of anticipation.

You know that all kinds of victories are going to be yours—victories you could never have realized had your life remained calm and on an even keel. Had there been no agonizing act of surrender, you could not have qualified for Nevertheless Living.

Oddly enough, the most desperate stage of depression, even suicidal thoughts, are "backed up" to Nevertheless Living. That is to say, they exist almost touching each other. But of course you don't know that until you enter Nevertheless Living. Unfortunately, there are no road signs along the way to encourage you. It is a terrifying route of total trust.

One afternoon when I was struggling and so desperate I didn't want to live, God seemed to show me a little mental picture. I immediately rejected it because it looked like a chart or graph. I detest such things because I don't understand them. I wanted to scream at God, "Don't show me some neat little picture; just make the pain stop!"

God is very patient. The picture didn't go away. In desperation, I peeked at it. Hurriedly, not understanding or liking it, I sketched the pesky little mental image. Then, sitting at my kitchen table, looking at my drawing, I gasped. Why had no one ever told me this?

You haven't been ready until now, a silent voice answered me.

The graph looked like a circle with a line down the center dividing it in two halves. On the right-hand side were five different stages of faith, with perfect faith (or Nevertheless Living) at the top right-hand side. On the top left-hand side was the terrifying stage of fear, suicidal thoughts, and total hopelessness. If the circle had been a clock, these stages would have been at either side of twelve noon.

Still thinking of the circle as a clock, I saw that my faith was usually at about 3:15 or 3:20. When I received the news about Jerry the clock read literally 3:17 p.m. That was when tragedy struck and my faith plunged to the bottom of the circle.

Knowing I should be at the top of the situation where Chris

FEAR-FAITH CIRCLE

A. CANNOT MOVE FROM *DEEP TRUST*, ETC. TO *NEVERTHELESS LIVING*. MUST MOVE TO THE RIGHT OR CUT ACROSS—SEE B.

B. MAY MOVE FROM ANY STAGE OF RIGHT HAND SIDE, I.E., *DOING FOR OTHERS*, TO ANY STAGE OF FEAR ON LEFT HAND SIDE, I.E., *MORBID NATURE (DEPRESSION)*, IN ONE STEP.

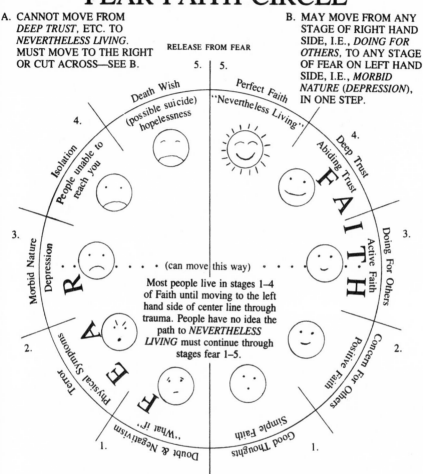

RELEASE FROM FEAR

Death Wish (possible suicide) hopelessness

Perfect Faith "Nevertheless Living"

Isolation

People unable to reach you

Abiding Trust

Deep Trust

Morbid Nature Depression

Active Faith

Doing For Others

Most people live in stages 1–4 of Faith until moving to the left hand side of center line through trauma. People have no idea the path to *NEVERTHELESS LIVING* must continue through stages fear 1–5.

· · · (can move this way) · · ·

Physical Symptoms

Terror

Positive Faith

Concern For Others

Doubt & Negativism "What if."

Simple Faith

Good Thoughts

BEGINNING OF FEAR

tians belong, I tried to climb back through the stages of faith (to the right). But that is not the way the clock of spiritual growth turns. I felt trapped as faith and fear battled one another in a crosscurrent at the bottom of the circle.

The only solution I found, in my exhaustion, was to cease all activity, relax, and let fear run its terrifying course (up the left side of the circle). By allowing fear to do all it could, I was letting fear defeat itself, although I didn't know it (and neither did the enemy). I was certain life would never again have meaning.

By letting fear do its worst, and still looking at the circle as a clock, I wound up at 11:55—the most desperate stage of fear.

Right next door, just a tiny step away, was sweet relief, even joy. Only no one had told me. I thought it was the end of everything, while actually I was only one step from Nevertheless Living!

Tragically, most people never make that one little step into victory, with the battle so nearly won. The traveler, devastated and terrified, is now ready to become more than a conqueror. The enemy wants to prevent us from taking that simple step of surrender, even though we are almost home free at Nevertheless Living.

The Nevertheless Principle explains how I took that step.

The
Nevertheless
Principle

1

The Long, Long Night

The night before Jerry's brain surgery were the most horrible hours of my life. While I lay on a little cot by my husband of almost twenty-five years in a hospital room in Decatur, Georgia, the spectre of *what-if* consumed me slowly, methodically.

Jennifer, our twenty-year-old daughter, was asleep on sofa pillows on the floor near my cot. I had not slept in three nights. Nor had I eaten in three days. When you are full of what-ifs, there is no room for anything else, not even a drink of water. As the nurses came in and out checking on Jerry, I realized that my mouth was unnaturally dry—partially from fear, but also from not even sipping liquid for so long. I lay on the cot dehydrated, defeated, terrified. Jerry slept soundly without even a sleeping pill, snoring slightly.

How ironic that the worst night of my life was in many ways the most wonderful of his! Christian friends had come by the room for prayer that evening. During that simple yet powerful prayer, Jerry had released himself totally to Jesus.

Facing brain surgery about which the doctors were not one bit optimistic, it seemed almost as though a light had gone on inside Jerry. He glowed. He couldn't stop smiling or talking about the reality of Jesus. He told the hospital maids about Jesus. The nurses. Everyone. He had the maids stand still, brooms in hand, while he read to them from his Bible. He had been set free from the fear of surgery and also from the fear of man and his opinions. It no longer mattered what people thought. Jerry wanted only to please God now. It was something I had longed for in his life since my own commitment to Jesus twelve years earlier.

He had new power right away. From his hospital bed despite the negative prognosis, he ministered to us, his family, and anyone who came into the room. As Jennifer and I helped him wash his hair with an antiseptic in preparation to have his head shaved for surgery, he sang and whistled his favorite hymns. One I remember was "Blessed Assurance." He even laughed and joked until Jennifer and I had to laugh, too. As scared as I was, he could make me laugh.

Laughter had always been part of Jerry's life. Julie, our married daughter, told me once, "I can't remember a day that Daddy wasn't smiling and laughing." Jerry's sense of humor had been the first thing I loved about him when we started to date. I would have married him just because of his dry, sharp sense of humor.

Of course, I soon learned to love many other qualities about him. Like his ability to see good in everyone. I didn't know what to call it back in the '50s, but I know now it was his spiritual gift of edification: he constantly built people up. I liked the way he never seemed to need attention in a crowd, but was content to remain in the background. Most of all I liked the way his eyes always laughed a few moments before a smile reached his mouth.

Now in this small room in DeKalb General Hospital, I suspected he was smiling even in his sleep. I lay motionless on the cot staring at the dimly lit ceiling. I had asked Jennifer to stay with me tonight because the fear battle was worst when Jerry was asleep and I was alone.

I could feel the fear moving around inside me, slowly but forcefully, like a full-term baby. Except it wasn't in my stomach, but in my chest. It stretched and kicked and elbowed me. People say "cold fear," but the kind I was experiencing was extremely hot. It pierced my ears like hot ice picks, formed a perfect square at the base of my neck, and a circle in the middle of my back. It was real and alive, moving around inside me and in the hospital room, too. My eyes burned from lack of sleep. I stood once to check on Jerry and nearly collapsed from fatigue. Fear is very tiring. The night seemed to last for weeks. How could one night be so long? "What if . . . ? What if . . . ?" crowded my mind as the hours crawled past.

What if it's malignant? What if they can't get it all? What if Jerry dies? What if I have to live a lifetime without him? What if I have to stand by and watch him suffer for months and months? What if there's no meaning to life anymore? What if the rest of my life is like tonight?

A nurse tiptoed in. "Are you asleep, Mrs. West? Need anything?"

"No," I replied quickly.

I longed to cry out, "I can't sleep. I'm too scared. Could you hold me a minute? Talk to me? Sit with me?" But I remained silent. The fear was so paralyzing I couldn't express it. No prayers that brought sweet relief welled up inside me. There wasn't room. The monster of fear was taking up all the room.

I knew Scripture. I knew how to pray. Why, I had written four books about my spiritual journey. I lectured and counseled about fear. I had lots of Christian friends, many of whom had been in this very room these past three days, praying with great faith. Our favorite Scriptures were taped to the walls. I had told countless others when in situations similar to mine, "Just quote Scripture. Stand on the Word. Jesus is the healer, the same yesterday, today and forever."

It was hard to breathe. My mouth was dry like cotton. I couldn't swallow. *Jennifer, please wake up. Hold me for a few minutes, please.*

I must have said the words aloud, because Jennifer's drowsy voice murmured, "Go to sleep, Mother. Stop wiggling and thinking."

You're alone, fear insisted. *What if you have to spend the rest of your life alone?*

O God, this can't be happening. Just a few weeks ago every-

thing was wonderful. Only . . . I didn't know how wonderful it was. Strange how we don't appreciate things until they're taken away.

This nightmare had begun six weeks ago on September 9, 1982. Jerry had taken off from work early that day because our fourteen-year-old son Jon was to be starting quarterback in a football game at his school. Jerry must have sensed something was wrong, though he said nothing, because to my astonishment he asked me to drive—a thing he had never done before.

On our way to the game we stopped at Jeremy's school to pick up our other son. (Although Jon and Jeremy are twins—because they *are* twins—the boys were attending different schools that year.) Driving on, with three of us in the car, I saw out of the corner of my eye that Jerry's head was tilted back, as though he were staring intently at something on the roof of the car.

I turned to look. His face was blue. Blood and saliva trickled from a corner of his mouth. The next moment he collapsed heavily against me.

How I got him to the hospital I'll never know. Blowing the horn with one hand, steering with the other, part of the way I drove over eighty miles an hour, with Jeremy crying, "Daddy! Daddy!" from the backseat.

The paramedics who hustled him from the car thought at first that he was dead. On the examining table, however, Jerry opened his eyes. "Have we missed the kickoff?" he asked. He felt so good that the doctor and I had to argue to keep him from getting up. Even as we remonstrated with him, another of the "seizures," as the doctor termed them, struck, turning his entire body rigid.

He recovered from this one just as swiftly, however, and although he was hospitalized five days and underwent every kind of test, including a CAT scan of the brain, doctors could not discover the cause.

How I now valued our life together! The things I had criticized him for no longer seemed important. So what if he was constantly late? I could learn to be late, too. So what if he wasn't outspoken like me and would rather make peace at any cost? The world needed peacemakers, and I could become quieter and stop crusading so much. I knew he thought I was a religious fanatic. Well, I could become a "normal" Christian. I knew he got upset when I mismatched his socks. (They all looked the same color to me.) I could take more time and do it right, and I could learn to work in the garden with him and not complain about shelling butter beans anymore. And I could start going fishing with him. I could even watch ball games on television.

After Jerry was released from the hospital, we enjoyed what is called "the good life"—for six weeks. We were in love again, almost as though we were dating! I had tried so often over the years to put the romance back into our marriage. Jerry would shrug his shoulders and pick up the sports page and put up with me, the way one does a chattering child.

"Jerry?" I would persist.

"Marion, what do you want me to do?" he would reply in exasperation.

"I want you to look at me when we talk, or just look at me. We don't really have to say anything, but let's just look at each other."

"Couldn't you say something sweet and warm?" I begged once.

He glared at me, then laughter sparkled in his blue eyes. "Hot chocolate chip cookies."

"That's not what I mean, Jer. You know it's not!"

"You think too much, Marion. Don't be so serious. We don't need to tell each other how we feel."

Now, after that stay in the hospital, I didn't have to encourage Jerry to communicate. I would catch him just staring at me. He started calling me the name he used when we were dating, *Mannie*. The TV set often went untouched now. "There's a football game on," I would call out.

"Who cares? Come sit by me, Mannie."

I would be there in an instant, and he would say, "I love you more than you can imagine."

That may not seem like a lot to many women, but expressions of love had not come easily for Jerry. He kept deep feelings to himself. Actually, we had gotten married without his ever saying, "I love you." Oh, he said it with his eyes, and in other ways—cards, letters—but never in the words I wanted to hear. Now we were communicating beautifully, finally, after almost twenty-five years!

He was more open with his love for the children, too. Even Jamie, our year-old granddaughter, noticed the change. She would run into his arms, whereas before Jerry's hospital stay she shied away from him.

For certain, there was something new and powerful between Jerry and Jesus. Not that he had just met Jesus. But there was something new and intimate in their relationship.

Now that idyllic six-week interval was about to come to a close. It was early morning. Jennifer was in her room. (She attended Mercer University in Atlanta and lived at home.) Jon and Jeremy had already left for high school. Jerry was getting ready for work. Something about the way he moved gave me an uneasy feeling. He walked slowly through the upstairs hall, looking into each bedroom almost as though he were a guest. I saw a puzzled look cross his face, as though he wasn't really certain which room was ours.

"I'm O.K., Mannie, really. Everyone gets a little confused at times." He was standing in the hall at the door of Jennifer's bedroom.

"Daddy?" Jennifer asked from inside the room. Her eyes met mine and we knew.

"I'm O.K., Jen," Jerry said. He was holding onto the door now.

"Come on, Jer." I touched his arm and directed him to our bedroom. I barely got him to the bed when I saw that look again—the same look I had seen in the car six weeks before. "Jerry, don't look at the wall like that," I screamed. "Please, Jerry."

"Daddy!" Jennifer cried, standing behind us. An unnatural

smile had inched across his face. He was staring at the wall as though he saw something we couldn't see. Then it hit, a massive seizure.

In the hospital the doctor had taught me how to prevent Jerry from biting his tongue in the event of a recurrence. Now I grabbed the gauze-wrapped tongue depressor from where I had hidden it in my dresser drawer and got it under his tongue in time. Meanwhile, Jennifer tried to reach the doctor by phone. The seizure passed, then another struck.

We couldn't reach the doctor for over two hours, although I did speak with the neurologist on call. The three of us stayed on the bed, soothing one another, even laughing some. Jerry insisted he was all right, but he couldn't sit up. He had almost no control over his body. Then a third seizure threatened.

"Daddy, you're not going to have another seizure," Jennifer said. "This is ridiculous.. It's not necessary."

"O.K., hon," he smiled. But his body started to twitch.

Shocked but encouraged by Jennifer's stand, I found a new supply of courage as we battled the renewed onslaught of seizures. "Sing, Jerry!" I urged. We all plunged into "Blessed Assurance."

"Look right into my eyes," I told him. He did and we sang and sang. Each time he let his eyes wander toward the wall, I commanded him almost sharply, "Jerry, look right into my eyes!" And we kept going like that, actually fighting off the seizures, until at last the doctor phoned.

I knew what the doctor would say and she did: Come to the hospital. By the time the ambulance arrived, Jerry was able to walk with help. We headed down the hall for the emergency room of DeKalb General once again. As before, Jerry was admitted to Intensive Care and the testing was repeated.

And still they could find nothing. The CAT scan looked normal. In a few days he was dismissed for the second time.

We didn't have so much joy this time as I drove him home. In fact, we had been home only a few hours when the call came. I answered the phone. The radiologist had reexamined the latest

CAT scan. There was something there after all. A mass, hopefully an abscess. Serious, but treatable with surgery and massive doses of antibiotics.

"I think we can help you," the neurologist, Dr. Loren, said, but there was caution in her gentle voice. She scheduled Jerry to reenter the hospital for brain surgery in three days.

But that same afternoon he began running a low-grade fever—a danger sign, we had been cautioned. I called Dr. Loren back: "I know it's your day off, but I'm begging you to admit him now. Please."

She didn't hesitate. "Leave for the hospital immediately. I'll have orders ready."

I draped a pair of new red pajamas over my arm, grabbed the car keys and my purse, and called out, "Come on, Jer." Someone else would have to figure out what else we needed at the hospital. Decisions were getting hard to make, even simple ones.

Finally we were through the ordeal of admittance once again. I was heading for Jerry's room with a bucket of ice when I met Dr. Loren in the hall. I hated what I saw in her eyes. "We suspect a massive tumor, but we could be wrong. The neurosurgeon will come by tomorrow to talk to you. I have to check on one more test and then I'll be on in."

I nodded. She probably guessed my face would give me away as soon as I saw Jerry. This way she wouldn't have to be the one to break it to him. I would have done the same thing in her place. I liked her a lot and so did Jerry.

"Hi." I walked into Jerry's room and set the ice down.

He was sitting on the side of his bed eating supper. He put his spoon down. "What is it?"

I picked up the spoon and began eating his chocolate pudding. What-ifs were attacking fiercely. There were no tears or tremors, just the hard, cold terror of what-if.

"What is it, Mannie?" Tears brimmed his eyes. No hint of laughter now.

I didn't know where to begin, but I knew I was going to begin. I loved him too much to just stand there silently. Dr. Loren had given me this opportunity. I took another spoonful of pudding, as if I could somehow get courage from it.

"Marion, are you just going to keep on calmly eating pudding?"

"They think the mass might be something more than an abscess. They won't know until surgery." It was my voice I heard, but I had no sense of having spoken. Everything seemed mechanical.

Jerry's job as health services manager at Georgia Power involved a lot of medical follow-up. Though his own degree was in electrical engineering, he did a great deal of work with doctors. He added up the score quickly. We stared at one another. Then he dropped his head and cried.

I couldn't cry. I remembered once I cut my hand so deeply that it didn't bleed for a long time. This slash in my life was too deep for tears. I just kept eating the chocolate pudding and watching Jerry. *Somehow*, I thought, *if I keep right on eating, everything will be all right again. Our world can't just fall apart while I'm standing here eating chocolate pudding.*

But what-ifs were coming hard and fast, as though I were being stoned to death. I simply let them strike me without even trying to shield myself. I felt numb, as if I had had a shot of Novocaine all over my body and into my spirit and mind. Reality seemed to be slipping away. In fact, my only link with the real world seemed to be the chocolate pudding and it was disappearing fast.

Jerry stopped crying and held out his arms to me. I went to him. Dr. Loren came in. She didn't stay long and she was crying as she left the room. I was grateful for her emotional involvement with us. So many doctors steel themselves not to feel. Dr. Loren, young, pretty, had jumped in with both feet and she was getting hurt. It helped some to have her hurt with us.

And now it was three nights later and I was tossing sleeplessly on my cot beside Jerry's hospital bed. Finally, oh, finally, the first hints of pink streaked through the dark sky. The morning of Jerry's brain surgery had arrived; the long, long night was almost over. Jerry and Jennifer still slept soundly. Now the day would begin, Monday, October 30, 1982. Jerry was really going to be rolled away for brain surgery and I was really going to sit and wait for the surgeon's report.

The small hospital room was filled with what-ifs. I wanted to open the window and order them all out. Looking back, I know now that I could have. But answers have never come easily for me. I was going to have to struggle through months of what-ifs before I found an answer.

Jerry, oh, Jerry, you are a part of me. Just like my arms and legs. I'm having brain surgery, too. Only they aren't putting me to sleep.

2

The Coat Rack

Jerry greeted the new day with smiles and encouraging words for everyone. When a lab technician had difficulty getting a blood sample—when her face flushed and she was obviously hurting Jerry and uncertain of her skills—he never stopped praising and encouraging her. *Leave him alone,* I wanted to scream, but I didn't want to start screaming; I might not be able to stop. "Please get your supervisor," I said in a controlled voice, and she left gratefully.

They didn't come to get Jerry for surgery until almost ten instead of the scheduled eight o'clock, so we endured more waiting. Outside in the hall, our friends and family and people from Jerry's office waited with us. For some reason, the nurses didn't ask them to clear the corridor. All the nurses liked Jerry's smile, his confidence, his sense of humor and his sincere interest in them. He absolutely refused to complain or say anything negative.

I kept listening for the sound of the stretcher wheels coming down the hall. I felt like a trapped animal. I detest hunting. I know all the arguments for hunting and trapping, but I've always wanted to run through the woods and loose everything caught. I even hate mousetraps. We had mice in the house once but I cried and begged Jerry not to buy a mousetrap. He didn't understand, but he didn't buy a trap and the mice disappeared. Now the jaws of anguish were clamped shut on me, and I understood why trapped animals often chewed their limbs off to be free.

The stretcher was coming. Jerry opened his arms to hold me. The orderlies stood waiting patiently. When we parted, Jerry was smiling. I almost envied his peace. "I'm going to be O.K., Mannie. Don't worry. See you in a little bit. I love you." His eyes held mine. It was the look I had longed for and nagged him for for almost twenty-five years.

I nodded silently and they rolled him away. I grabbed his extended hand and walked alongside him; many of our friends and family followed. We were a long procession going down the hall to the elevator. Jerry looked radiant. Jesus' joy was all over him. As the doors shut on the elevator, he called out, "Keep the faith, Mannie."

We had to vacate his room; after surgery he would be taken to Intensive Care. Some friends began gathering up our things. The neurosurgeon had told me that the longer it took the better: it meant they were getting it. I stumbled into the waiting room. It was crowded with friends and family, so many that some had to stand. Jerry's mother and dad were there. My mother. Our daughter Julie, and her husband, Ricky; Jon, Jeremy and Jennifer. All the people dearest to me in the world—except one.

Suddenly I couldn't bear for anyone to look at me. There was a small metal coat rack in the corner. I got a sheet from one of the nurses, hung it over the rack, and crawled inside the makeshift tent. I didn't care what anyone thought. Nothing was real anyway. I curled up in a fetal position, shaking hard.

People kept sticking food behind the sheet. I couldn't eat. I still couldn't even sip water. I was packed full of what-ifs. *This can't be happening,* I thought. *We were living a happy, normal life. Jerry was the picture of health. He's never once taken sick leave from work in twenty-five years.*

I came out of my tent long enough to ask to see Jerry's room in the Intensive Care unit. "Of course," the nurse smiled. Too nice. Everyone was being too nice. I followed her down the hall.

Jo Ann Thomason, one of my dearest friends, saw what was happening and got up and went with me. She was crying. I still couldn't cry.

"This is where he will come, Mrs. West. Right here by the nurses' station where we can take really good care of him."

I knelt down by the bed. Three hot tears slid down my face and spotted the sterile covers. I put my head down and whispered, "Please, God, oh, please. I'll do anything, anything. Pay any price. Please, please, please . . . even if he's disabled for life. That's O.K. Just let him live. I can take care of him."

Jo Ann stood in a corner and cried.

Back in the waiting room we waited some more. I hid in my tent cubicle. I had just come out to stretch my legs when the nurse came in. "Dr. Long wants to talk to you, Mrs. West, and all the immediate family." The jaws of the trap tightened. The doctor should have come to the waiting room. What if . . . ?

I followed the nurse, along with the rest of the family. We entered a conference room and sat at a long, shiny table as though we were at a house closing. Dr. Long came in, dressed in a neat business suit. Like the excellent surgeon he was, he cut through to the truth. Deep and clean. No superficial little stabs.

"He came through the surgery fine. The tumor, however, is highly malignant, the worst possible kind. Astrocytoma grade-four, glioblastoma, multi-form. I could remove only part of it. Nothing will make any difference. If I had operated on day one, it still would not have helped. However, I will recommend cobalt to begin within a few days. He has a few months at most."

It was as though the doctor had drawn an invisible machine gun and methodically riddled bullets through us. One by one a family member screamed or sobbed or fell onto the table. All except Julie and me. I remember sitting very erect, staring at the second hand on the wall clock. It was 3:17, then 3:18. The doctor talked on for ten minutes or so, but I heard nothing else.

That's the kind of clock that was in the delivery room when our children were born, I thought. I felt as though I had literally turned to stone. Very cold and hard—as though the blood had stopped circulating. They said that I turned completely white. *I will not crumble at this doctor's words. There must be a way out of this.*

One by one the family left the room. Someone led me out, too. I was thinking, *I wish the doctor had still been in his operating clothes. I wish he'd been sweaty, even bloody. I wish his voice had broken just once*—even though I understood that a surgeon could not do what he had to do, day in and day out, if he allowed himself the luxury of breaking down.

In Intensive Care Dr. Loren was waiting. "When he gets here, we'll have to tell him—either me or Dr. Long."

"No! I want to tell him in my own way. Please give us some time alone."

"All right. But one of us will have to talk to him, too."

Jennifer arrived. "Mama, I just saw Daddy coming down the hall from surgery! He said, 'Hey, sugar.' He looks great."

Within a matter of minutes they had him in bed, looking marvelous with a neat bandage around his head. His shaved hair was in a plastic bag; I quickly threw it in the trash can.

"Hey, love," I said, sitting on the bed.

"Hiedy."

It was a word I first heard him use in high school. It meant much more than hello. It meant, "Well, hello there. I like you. We're going to have some good times." It was the word he used when calling from out-of-town, the one he used after each of our children was born. It was a wonderful, special word.

Jerry glanced at the calendar. "The date's wrong. Fix it."

"What difference does it make?"

Then I remembered. When testing brain function, doctors use questions like *What date is it?* or *Who's the President?*

"The calendar says the 29th," Jerry pointed out. "It's the 30th."

I tore off a page and Jerry grinned.

I took a deep breath. "They couldn't get it all," I said, "but cobalt treatments should help, and of course we have Jesus, the Healer."

"Right," he kept smiling.

Dr. Loren came in. She squeezed Jerry's toe, sat at the foot of the bed and kept patting his foot. She said how good he looked and then somehow worked in that all his affairs should be put in order. I didn't hear the word *malignant*. She left abruptly, tears welling up in her eyes.

Our children gathered around the bed. Jeremy had a present for his father, a fancy screwdriver. On the box was printed *The master's tool.*

O God, don't use Jerry in some marvelous way that requires taking him! Leave him here and use him.

Jerry opened the box. "Hey, Jeremy, thanks, son," he beamed.

"It's for when you come home and fix things again," Jeremy explained.

"I really like it."

While the rest of the family came in for short visits, the what-ifs started inside me again. *What if you have to live without him?* I simply couldn't, that was all. Whenever Jerry had had a business trip, he waited until the last possible moment to tell me. I always hit rock bottom when I knew he had to be gone, even for one night. No, I could not live without him. There would be no reason to get up or dress or put on makeup or set the table or plant flowers. There would be no more laughter or joy or love . . . no one to say *hiedy.*

Already the fear of our house without Jerry had taken hold of me and I knew I couldn't go home to sleep. I couldn't turn in our driveway or go up those steps, past the roses Jerry had planted for one of our anniversaries. I couldn't even see our collie. Someone else would have to figure out what to do about the children and food. I realized that I was walking a beaten, humble walk, not straight and tall, and I started to whisper when I spoke.

I accepted Charlie and Dru Glisson's invitation to go home with them for a few days—they included the boys, too. At their house, Dru ran me a bath, laid out a pink gown and made some tea.

"He's going to be all right, Marion," Charlie said. "God's going to heal him."

"What?"

"Jerry's going to be all right. The doctors are wrong."

I loved those words and the way Charlie smiled when he said them. I looked at Dru and whispered, "I can't sleep alone."

I wanted to stop whispering, but couldn't seem to get my normal voice back. *Others have gone through this,* I thought. *God, how did they do it?*

"I'll sleep in the guest room," Charlie laughed. "You sleep with Dru." I was glad he was laughing. It sounded so good in a world where nothing seemed normal anymore.

In the bed, what-ifs intensified. A hot circle and square of fear were burning on my back again. "Dru, it's like a living thing, the fear."

She placed her hand where the fear sat and began to pray softly. "For tonight, Marion, I'm going to ask God to put all your feelings on me. I'll stay awake and pray. You sleep. He will give you sweet sleep."

And He did. I couldn't even worry about Dru staying awake and praying for me. But morning brought that intense fear again. I forced myself to get up. Someone had brought me clothes. It must have been Jennifer because everything matched and was color-coordinated. Dru and Charlie drove me to the hospital. We had to stop by my house for something, I can't remember what. Dru went inside while I hid my face in my hands. I was afraid of my own driveway and front yard. *What if Jerry never pulls in here at six o'clock anymore? What if we can't rake leaves together next fall? What if the dogwood blooms without him?*

As we backed out of the driveway, I told God, *I can't live without him. You need to understand that. I can't any more than I could breathe under water. I grew up without a daddy and I can't grow old without a husband. I won't.*

It was a clear, sunny day in early fall. Usually we would be planning a football game. As we drove to the hospital, I ran back mentally into a world of memories. I tried to gather and salvage days, feelings, emotions—hold onto them, store them away. I ran as though hot lava were on my heels. I had to gather up in my arms all the wonderful, funny, not-so-funny memories of a life-time, before they were snatched away. Memories of Jerry happy and healthy, swimming, playing football, mowing the grass, planting his garden. . . .

Don't let go! Hold on! something inside me kept screaming. It never occurred to me that victory might lie in exactly the opposite direction. But letting go never once entered my mind.

3

Voices

Jerry came home from the hospital on the fifth day after surgery. We went shopping for hats for him the next day. Friends we happened to meet couldn't believe how good Jerry looked, or that we were actually out shopping.

He was different from the old Jerry in so many ways. One day while we were eating out, a waitress behaved in an unbelievably lewd fashion, much to the delight of the male customers. Jerry called her over and she came laughing, expecting him to encourage her. In a gentle voice he said, "Young lady, you have been deceived by Satan. He's having a heyday with you. Please don't talk like that anymore." She quieted down in a hurry, while the laughing men looked seriously at their food. The old Jerry would never have risked a public scene.

Before one of our boys' football games, one of the players started using four-letter words to his mother, doing it in a loud voice so that many people heard. The mother stood like a statue, as though it were a common occurrence. Jerry walked over to the boy, put his hands on his shoulders and looked him squarely in the eyes: "Son, don't ever speak to your mother that way again. Satan has a grip on you. You need God in your life." And to the astonished woman he said, "You must put a stop to that kind of

talk now." The Jerry I used to know would never have inter-
fered.

We held hands everywhere we went now. Jerry smiled almost
constantly. But early mornings were extremely hard for him. He
would wake up crying uncontrollably. Within a few minutes he
would confess the fear and self-pity as sin, ask forgiveness and
receive instant relief. But it was terrifying to me that when he
cried, I froze. I couldn't seem to feel anything anymore. I would
watch him, wanting to help, but I was so needy myself that I
simply could not respond. It was as though my tear ducts had
been removed. Throughout the entire ordeal I cried only three
brief times. Sometimes I envied Jerry because he could cry.

I grieved. Grieved as though he were gone. I recalled a poem
I had written in high school for no particular reason. I had had no
specific person in mind. Only the first few lines came back, but
they were enough to intensify my agony.

The Year After You Were Gone

Spring came again this year . . .
I knew it would . . .
And yet I wondered how it could.
But it came all green and pink and white . . .
Bringing sweet perfume that spilled into the night.

I had not thought of that poem in almost twenty-nine years.
Now it played over and over in my mind like a stuck record. My
mind, in fact, was filled with voices over which I seemed to have
no control. *You can write a book,* they suggested. *You can call it*
A World Without Jerry. *That's a good title.*

But a world without Jerry would be no world at all for me.
Anyhow, I was certain I would never write again. What did I
have to share? I was totally defeated by fear. I phoned *Guideposts*
and asked permission to back out of a contract to provide thirty
devotionals for *DAILY Guideposts 1984.* I had submitted only

half that number. The editors were very concerned about Jerry and graciously told me not to worry about the remaining fifteen pieces.

I became almost physically sick every evening about six. That had been Jerry's coming-home time. I used to sit in a chair in the living room by the window and watch for his car. If I wasn't busy, sometimes I would watch for over an hour—a habit I had formed in childhood when I watched for Mother to come home from work. Even when I wasn't by the window, I could hear the car above the other sounds in our noisy home. It didn't matter whether Jerry and I were on especially good terms; my heart would still leap when I heard his car turn into the driveway. The voice now insisted, *He won't be coming home anymore. What will you do?*

When we lived in Macon before the twins were born, Jerry got a promotion, which meant moving to Athens. He took a motel room there, intending to come home on weekends, while I was to remain in our house in Macon until it sold. At six each evening I stood at the window in Macon believing somehow that he would come home, even though I knew he was in Athens. When Jerry called each night, all I did was cry. After five days he came and got Julie and Jennifer and me. We moved into an old house in Athens that was totally inadequate and lived there until the Macon house sold and we could build a new one. I never complained; my husband was home in the evenings.

Now, although Jerry was right there at home recuperating from his surgery, I would watch the clock for six to come. When it did, I was unable to keep from going to the living room window and looking out. *He's sitting down in the den,* I would try to reason with myself. *Why are you looking out the window?* The voices would reply, *You're trying to see what it will feel like when he isn't coming home anymore. You need to do this.*

I looked out, watching, hurting, terrified of the cars moving past our house. They all had husbands in them. Then I went back and looked down the five steps from the kitchen to where Jerry was sitting on the sofa in the den. "See, he's right there," I would whisper to myself. "There's no need to look out the window."

Inevitably though, I would walk back to the window, my fear taking over. *There's no possible way I can live without him,* I told God again. *I can't live for my children, or to write. It's not enough. He is my world. I'm sorry. I know that's not right, but he is.*

It wasn't exactly like praying. God seemed far away. I was used to His being so close that I could touch Him. Now the terrifying voices seemed to be all I could hear.

I had to do all the driving now. And sometimes when I was alone in the car, the voices would show me a certain curve and point out, *If you went very fast around this curve, you could end it all. You could get relief. You know you can't live without him. Even if you weren't killed, you'd get to go to the hospital and they'd give you something and you wouldn't have to make decisions anymore.*

I always made myself reduce my speed until I crept along the expressway with everyone passing me. But I would imagine myself speeding around the curve. . . .

Thanksgiving came. Somehow I had thought maybe it wouldn't, this year. Our families came and cooked and brought food and we did all the traditional things. I had lost fifteen pounds in the less-than-a-month since the tumor was discovered and could not eat. I didn't think I would ever eat again. Sometimes I wondered if I would ever laugh again. Or even smile. Sometimes when I was out at the store, I looked at women alone, wondering if they were widows, and I watched to see if they ever smiled. How could they?

Jerry and I went to a Christian luncheon at someone's home. A young widow was there, Penny De Haan. She had lost two husbands on the same date nine years apart in plane crashes. Her second husband, Dan, had been a well-known Bible teacher and author. He had been flying home from a Bible conference less than a year before when the crash had occurred. Penny wore an attractive dress, perfect makeup, talked about her children . . . and laughed.

At the lunch table someone asked her something. A look of absolute delight crossed her face as she said softly, "I'm a vessel for the Lord now. He can do whatever He chooses with me."

God, I thought, *don't ask me to be a vessel! I'm a wife. I've done it all wrong for almost twenty-five years, made so many mistakes. I've nagged Jerry about surrendering everything to You. But see, he's done it now. And I know how to be a wife. I really do. We're in love. Look at us. Surely You can see how in love we are. Don't ask me to become a vessel. I will only be a wife. You have to let me be a wife now that I know how.*

After lunch the Bible study started. Jerry tapped me on the shoulder, asking as a small child might have asked how to find the passage in the Bible. I tried to brush away the fear that knotted my stomach and found the page for him.

Later we had a magnificent prayer time for Jerry. The couple in whose home we were meeting had a real prayer closet with a stained glass window. We all gathered in there and prayed for Jerry, thanking God for his healing. I opened my eyes to look at him. He was positively glowing, as though a light had switched on inside him. *See,* I told myself, hoping the menacing voices would hear, *everything's going to be all right. So what if he got confused looking up Scripture? He's had lots of cobalt.*

Night after night I prayed after Jerry was asleep. I would reach over and go up and down his body with my hand, praying for total healing, quoting Scripture. Sometimes I prayed half the night. Other times I knelt beside him on the bed and prayed while he was awake. Often the children gathered around and we all prayed, or friends came in to pray with us. We confessed sin, forgave each other, made everything right between us and everyone we knew.

But no matter what I did, or what Jerry did, each morning it was the same for me. Just as I was coming out of sleep, before I was even half-awake, the voices (there were always more in the morning) were waiting for me with a message that never changed: *Your husband is dying. Your husband is dying. . . .*

4

A Shawl for Thelma

At the time I didn't know what to call it. Looking back, I know it was my first taste of Nevertheless Living and it happened, of all places, in the radiation wing of the hospital.

Jerry had begun cobalt therapy on November 10, eleven days after his surgery. I almost envied him as we awaited his turn for radiation. He walked in chipper and spoke to everyone in the waiting room. Sometimes he forgot to remove the warm fur hat we had bought after his head was shaved. In his medical folder was a photograph of him on the day treatment began. Smiling, wouldn't you know. Having a picture made for radiation therapy and he smiled as though it were a picture for the school annual.

After the nurse called him in for treatment, I would sit like a piece of stone, staring straight ahead, not wanting to speak to anyone. And it was there in the waiting room that God spoke to me.

It seemed I hadn't heard from Him in a long time, but I hadn't really been listening. What could He possibly say now?

Marion, the silent words formed in my heart, *I want you to go to the woman in the hall and speak to her about Me. She's in a wheelchair. You'll know the one I mean.*

I glanced into the hall and saw her—elderly, frail, clutching the sides of her wheelchair. Most of her hair was gone and she had that gaunt, hopeless look.

I don't want to, God. No use trying to pretend with Him. *I don't care about her. She's old. What about Jerry and me?*

Obey Me. I know what's best for you.

She's not going to respond. Look at her. She doesn't even care.

Go on, Marion. Tell her that I love her.

It was one of the most difficult things I had ever done, and I had done some pretty hard things lately. I walked over.

"Hi. My name's Marion. What's yours?"

She didn't respond. She looked straight ahead. I knew the feeling.

Keep trying.

"God loves you."

Her cold blue eyes met mine. "I don't believe in God."

I wasn't surprised, but something stirred within me. I was beginning to care about her, just a little. It felt good.

"He loves you anyhow. What's your name?"

"Thelma. I'm dying, you know. I've never believed in God or asked Him for anything and I'm too old and stubborn to start now."

"I like you," I almost smiled.

"Why?" she gasped.

"You're honest. I like honest people. See you tomorrow, O.K.?"

She nodded.

That night in bed I thought about Thelma again. Jerry was asleep. *Take her something.* Once more the thought was not my own. I began to think about what I could take. A Bible, a statue of praying hands?

No, no, God seemed to interrupt. *You don't take someone who doesn't believe in Me something like that.* Then He gave me explicit instructions. *Look up on the closet shelf, 'way back in the left-hand corner. Get the beautiful handmade shawl. Give that to Thelma and say, "This isn't a shawl. It looks like a shawl, but*

it's not. It's the arms of God loving you." Tell her it's from Me.
Then wrap the shawl around her with your arms and hold her a
little longer than necessary.

I hadn't seen the shawl in a year. Messy shelves have never bothered me and Jerry had learned to put up with my side of the closet. I could hardly believe the shawl would be there. I tiptoed across the room in the dark and reached up on the shelf. My hand went right to the soft material and I pulled it out in amazement. It was good to be communicating with God again.

The next day at therapy, Thelma was in the line again awaiting her turn—though as an in-patient she could have been brought down to the radiation wing at any time during the day. Standing behind her wheelchair, I pulled the shawl from the bag and placed it around her thin shoulders. I did it slowly and deliberately and enfolded her in my arms . . . a little longer than necessary.

"It's not from me. It's from God. Now, it may look like a shawl, but it's not." I waited.

"Well, what in the world is it, then?" Already she was stroking it as one would a kitten.

"It's the arms of God holding you and loving you." I walked around to face her. She stared at me, her mouth a small, round *o*. "Thelma, He loves you so much. Let Him into your heart!"

"But I've been so stubborn, for so long."

"Doesn't matter. He sent you the shawl."

At that moment an orderly arrived to wheel her to the treatment room, and Jerry came out walking that unsteady walk caused by radiation directly to the brain. I had to go to him.

Weeks passed. Jerry finished his treatment, and I never saw Thelma again. A close friend of mine, Rose McKeever, worked on the oncology floor. I learned from Rose that Thelma had not been a model patient. But one day she returned to her room from radiation therapy wearing a beautiful shawl and insisting that some strange woman had given it to her. Reports were that she was never without the shawl. Rose told me that Thelma began to smile and attend chapel and tell people that God loved them.

Thelma died two months later with the shawl wrapped around her, like the loving arms of God.

As I say, it was a foretaste of Nevertheless Living. But I had months of misery to endure before I would be ready for more.

5

The Christmas Tree

There was nothing I could do to stop Christmas from coming. Jerry was to have that week off from cobalt treatment. After his last session before the holidays, the doctor gave him and each of his patients a potted poinsettia plant to take home. Outside the hospital in the cold air, Jerry wasn't sure where the car was. I had to help him into the passenger seat.

I couldn't buy presents. The children kept insisting that I go Christmas shopping, or at least tell them what to buy. I just stared through them as though I didn't understand the language they were speaking.

"Can we have a tree?" Jeremy asked.

"No," I almost shouted. "No tree. I won't ever have a tree in this house again." So often Jerry and I had quarreled over the tree. . . .

One time when Julie was a baby, he had insisted we go out to the country and cut our own tree, like when he was a boy. I had forgotten Julie's bottle and she was screaming as Jerry drove slowly down a wooded lane. "We could have bought a tree for what the ax cost," I grumbled, jiggling Julie. Suddenly he saw the one he wanted, parked the car and got out. He was about to start cutting when an irate elderly man appeared and informed us that this was all private property. So we had a store-bought tree anyhow.

Jerry always wanted me to whip up soap powder and put it on our tree to look like snow, as his mother did when he was a boy in Galax, Virginia. I always refused to do it. Oddly enough, just the past Christmas, Jennifer had done it for him. He had sat and looked at the result with great satisfaction: "Now that's a tree!"

Now, this horrible Christmas, while I was out for a little while at the grocery store, the children put up a tree. I wouldn't even look at the loathsome thing. A friend brought us new red placemats, very cheery. I finally managed to put them on the table, but it was as though they weighed a hundred pounds each. I hung our traditional wreath on the door; even that simple action required energy and courage I didn't know I possessed.

I made countless trips to the drugstore to get prescriptions filled for Jerry. I would stand in line staring grimly ahead while people chattered and Christmas music filled the store. I had to walk past the gift wrap to the prescription counter, feeling as though I were walking on hot coals. I watched husbands hold open doors for wives whose arms were filled with packages. I watched fathers talking to children and listened as women told each other what they were getting their husbands. I almost gasped with pain when I walked by the card counter and saw the section marked *Season's Greetings: Husbands.*

Christmas hit Jerry especially hard, too. Usually he was bright and encouraging, but one evening he said, "Let's go for a ride, Mannie. I need to get out." We wrapped up and I got Jerry settled and then slid behind the wheel. I drove around and around. A steady rain was falling. Even the windshield wipers seemed to insist, *You're scared. You're scared.* We looked at the lights in happy homes.

Then Jerry began to cry. I still couldn't cry. I just had a dry ache that was the deepest pain I had ever known. Finally I pulled into a shopping center and parked. We watched people laughing, running, shopping, while Jerry's muffled crying filled the car. Just four months ago—less than that, I thought—we were like those people. Illness was totally foreign to us. O God, why couldn't we go back? I'd never fuss again. I'd put soap on the tree.

I got out of the car and went into a drugstore and bought Jerry some mints. His mouth was always dry from the medicine he was taking. I drove to our house three times and each time Jerry said, "I can't go in yet." The fourth time he was smiling that wonderful smile we all depended on, and I turned into the driveway.

The only shopping I had done was to buy sheets to fit the hospital bed we had gotten for him. He wasn't using it yet, but we got it ready downstairs in our recreation room.

It rained for three solid weeks that December. One morning we made a great effort and drove to church in the pouring rain. Just Jerry and me; the children stayed at home with their grandparents. On the carport were mounds of dead and dying worms. They always got swept on the carport when we had too much rain. We had to step on them to get into the car. Suddenly I knew how they felt. I hadn't seen anything in this nightmare that I could identify with, except the worms. I looked at them a long time. Jerry sometimes talked about my doing a book. "Put today in the book, Mannie, and be sure and tell how much it rained, O.K.?"

I received my *DAILY Guideposts, 1983* in the mail. I had written some of the devotionals, back when things were good . . . before I knew what it was to hurt like this, each moment of the day and night. Usually when I got my *DAILY Guideposts* I read straight through the year in a couple of sittings. This time I couldn't make myself look at the coming months. Someone gave me a beautiful Scripture calendar. I couldn't turn past January. I didn't want to see the future in print.

I finally agreed to let the children pick out a red and navy blue running suit for Jerry from me, and a doll for our granddaughter, Jamie. I remember that Jerry loved the running suit. He put it on after Christmas and said, "I'm going to do push-ups. You'll see." I was having to walk everywhere with him now. He'd fallen in the shower and cut his hand and there'd been several other falls. I had safety bars put up in the bathroom and determined to watch him more closely.

The doctor prescribed a brace for his left foot to keep it from dragging. He'd lost the use of his left hand completely. Still, he insisted upon dressing himself, although it took him almost an hour. Sometimes for hours he'd practice tying his shoes with one hand. "I can do it," he'd tell me, like a small, determined child.

Reluctantly I agreed to go to a Christmas party at church. I knew the moment we walked into that festive room that I shouldn't have come. I fixed Jerry's plate, but didn't touch my own food. Just stared ahead, panic rising in me. The voices were louder than ever: *This is your last Christmas with your husband. Aren't you going to sing "Silent Night"?*

Several close friends came by to ask if I was O.K. I shook my head, no. I felt as though I were being devoured by . . . something hard to define . . . maybe piranha, the vicious little fish that destroy you bit by bit. Several people prayed for me on the spot. I didn't feel any different.

Back at home, our friend Caryl Swift, who'd driven Jerry and me to the party, helped me get him upstairs. Then the three of us knelt by our bed and prayed for a long time. Afterward, Jerry was smiling joyously. I wanted to smile. I'd just forgotten how. I was afraid for Caryl to leave.

I wanted someone to hold onto, emotionally. I couldn't lean on Jerry now. I'd written a book called *Learning to Lean*, explaining how we must lean on Jesus. Why wasn't I doing it now?

You're a Christian, the voices mocked. *Where's your victory?*

I thought of a formula that had always worked for me in the past. No matter what is taken away from you, if you keep your eyes on Jesus and praise Him, He will restore it to you. You will be joyful to the exact same degree you have hurt. What you have lost will be replaced . . . joy for mourning . . . beauty for ashes. . . .

I walked to the door with Caryl. I almost wanted to scream, *Take me with you, don't leave me here!* And yet, nothing could have made me leave Jerry even for an instant. *What about your formula?* the voices gloated.

Standing alone at the foot of the steps as she drove off, I prayed, "God, I don't see how it could possibly work now. I don't see how You will ever come to me again in any shape or form. But I won't limit You, so I'm going to remember this moment for the rest of my life. And if and when You restore the years that the locusts have eaten, I will tell people about it and write about it. I am committing to You to remember this agony and if You can come up with some kind of joy to the equivalent that I hurt, You are truly a God of miracles."

I turned to go upstairs to help Jerry get ready for bed. As I started up the steps, I noticed that the lights on the Christmas tree were still on. I still hadn't looked directly at it. For twenty-four years, Jerry had always unplugged the Christmas tree lights each night. I walked over to the tree and looked at it for the first time. I squinted my eyes like a little girl trying to see how pretty I could make the lights.

Even with my eyes squinted the tree was not beautiful. There was no beauty anywhere this Christmas.

6

Nowhere to Run

In bed, after I'd turned off the tree lights, the what-ifs started again. They seemed to come out of the woodwork at night. To escape them I forced my mind back to my childhood. Swimming, favorite pets, Gene Autry, paper dolls, camp, trips, spend-the-night parties. I thought of a special girlfriend, Keith. We went all the way through school together and even roomed together at college. Suddenly a forgotten memory came vividly alive.

I was at her birthday party—we were maybe eight or nine. We had on pastel dresses with big sashes and ribbons in our hair. I had carefully asked her ahead of time, "Will your daddy be at your party?"

She replied, "No, he'll be at work. But he can see my presents when he gets home."

Immediate relief. Keith's daddy wouldn't be there. I would go. No one knew, but I didn't go to anyone's house if her daddy would be present. It reminded me that I didn't have one. At least I'd never known him: I wasn't quite two when he died of strep throat just before penicillin was available in 1938.

Sometimes I'd been at a friend's house, after ascertaining—seemingly casually—that her daddy was out of town. Then he'd appear after all, and I'd always figure out an excuse to leave. No one suspected. It wasn't that I wanted to avoid men. Several wonderful men whose children were grown lived in our neighborhood, and I always felt comfortable around them. I just didn't want to see any little girls with their daddies.

Knowing Keith's father wouldn't be at home, I went to her house full of the usual party excitement. We were all in her yard playing, when her daddy drove up unexpectedly. Keith screamed, "He came home!" He got out of the car and she ran into his arms. I didn't look. She dragged him over to me, holding his hand. "Look, Marion, Daddy got to come home for the party."

"Um, I don't feel too good. I think I have to go home." I ran all the way, blinking hard, so I wouldn't cry.

All my life, I thought, lying in bed beside my husband, I'd run away emotionally from situations that threatened me. *You grew up without a father,* the voices reminded me. *What if you have to grow old without a husband? What if you have to watch everyone march by, two by two, and you are all alone?*

Fear twisted around in my stomach. I could feel it moving. I tossed restlessly trying to wake Jerry up. A song Keith had danced to in a recital one time was spinning around in my head: "Two by two, they go marching through . . . Sweethearts on Parade. . . ."

Jerry woke up. "What's wrong, Mannie?"

"Make a big C."

It was a habit of almost twenty-five years. Sometimes he'd ask me first, "Make a little C." It was a comforting position where he curled around me. He made a big C and I held his hand in the dark. "Go to sleep," he mumbled gently. "Everything's O.K."

All January Jerry's health went downhill rapidly. Then, having lost the use of his left side, he made a miraculous, almost-overnight recovery. His left hand opened and he regained full use of it. We threw away the brace and he began doing push-ups and jogging in place.

Jerry was the only one who wasn't surprised. He'd never been one to get discouraged. I remembered how he used to head out for the golf course in the pouring rain. "Be reasonable, Jerry," I'd beg. "You can't play in this."

"Just a spring shower. It'll stop."

We were sure the recovery was the result of all the prayers that had been offered up for Jerry. *Guideposts* readers from all over the country and beyond wrote assuring us of their prayers. Many churches prayed.

The amazed doctors insisted that they'd never seen a hand open once it shut. One day coming home from church we pulled into a filling station and Jerry got out and pumped the gas himself. Another day we stopped to pick up some fried chicken and Jerry crossed Ponce de Leon Avenue by himself to use the restroom. "You're going by yourself," I called to him, joyfully.

"Yes, I'm a big boy now."

I began to notice men lifting things. I'd always taken such matters for granted. Now I stopped and stared as trash collectors heaved heavy loads onto trucks. I wanted to cry to them, "Do you know what a gift health is? Your mind and body working together beautifully? Have you thanked God?"

Even when a man did some small thing, like count correct change, I marvelled. I'd look at his head and think, *Everything is working properly inside there. What a miracle.* Sometimes the man would catch me staring and I'd have to look away. I wanted to look him in the eye and say, "Go home and love your wife tonight."

One night Jerry brought in wood for the fire and I praised God all evening. Another time I saw him throw a football to Jon and watched in open fascination, remembering the days I used to resent his playing ball with the twins, feeling myself neglected.

One day Jerry put on his new red and navy blue running suit and insisted that I take him to the track at the high school. While other men jogged around and around, Jerry walked, concentrating on each step. As the runners sped past him, he plodded along, stumbling a little, putting one foot in front of the other. When he finally got back to the starting point he was beaming. "Did you see me?"

I nodded. "You were marvelous. Ready to go home now?"

"No, I'm going to do it again. Watch me."

The doctors had said that he couldn't return to work, but he did. He refused Social Security and no one knew how to react to that. Seemed no one had ever refused it before. I had to learn to drive downtown to his office. Gone were the days when I said, "I can't." Letting Jerry out of the car in that traffic, knowing he was going in to compete with men who had no limitations, was the hardest thing I'd done yet.

"I have to go to work, Marion," he'd say. I knew he wanted to prove he could still work, but he was also concerned about us financially. His job was stressful and demanding, and looking back, I realized symptoms of the tumor had showed up there first, even before the first seizure. Sometimes there'd been a look in his eyes when he came home. I'd meet him at the door. "Have a good day?"

He'd kiss me, but he'd look . . . confused for a moment—almost alarmed—and very, very tired. "I can't catch up," he'd say. Then the look would pass and he'd start roughhousing with the boys, and I'd decide my imagination was working overtime.

One time before he got sick, I got up at three-thirty A.M. to find him still working on a budget. It was spread all over the floor. The words shot through my mind, *Something is wrong, very wrong.* A man shouldn't work twelve hours a day and then come home and work all night and still be behind. The work seemed to be too difficult suddenly. But I pushed those thoughts away. Jerry always said I went looking for things to worry about.

Now each time I let him out at work I had to fight the panic that rose up in me. *Oh, God, why does he have to push himself like this? He could walk out in front of a car, or have a seizure on the steps, or get lost or confused . . . or anything.* I'd drive home, make myself wait an hour or so and then phone. When he answered the phone, I wanted to crawl through it to him. "Hi!" I'd try to sound casual. "How's it going?"

"O.K.," but his voice told me different.

Some days all the way to work, he went over and over his appointment book, trying to get straight what he had to do that day. One time I insisted that we make an unscheduled stop at Dr.

Loren's. She examined him and announced, ''He looks great. No
reason he can't go to work.'' Clinically he passed every test.
What she didn't know was that he practiced them at home for
hours. I thought sometimes I'd scream if he didn't stop touching
the end of his nose with his index fingers. He was having trouble
telling time too, but I didn't tell the doctor. I could not betray
him. So I drove him to work, thinking: *I can do it one more day.*
I'll just do it today.

I did it for four months.

As I let him out one time, I noticed he'd lost so much weight
that his clothes weren't fitting right. And he was walking that
unsteady walk again. I had taken him to another building this day
for an important meeting. ''Bye, I'm fine,'' he insisted, smiling
as always. Looking in the rearview mirror, I could tell that he
didn't know for certain where the front door was. *Oh, God, what*
do You want me to do? People at work won't say anything,
they're too kind. All of them, the doctors and the people he
worked with, had told me they were depending on me to tell them
when I thought something was wrong. Something was terribly
wrong, but Jerry wanted so desperately to keep his job. *How*
much longer do You want me to do this, God? I feel like I'm
losing the ability to make rational decisions.

From the sidewalk Jerry turned around and waved. I waved
back and drove away.

7

Jerry's Job

I used to wonder when I was in school how soldiers could possibly keep walking when their feet were frozen. The pictures in our history books showed George Washington's troops, staggering through the snow looking as though they couldn't possibly take another step. Yet the books recorded that they marched on for miles and days. How could they have?

At last I understood. You just keep taking one more step . . . doing one more thing. Keeping on keeping on, even though everything inside is dead. *How can I possibly be buying groceries?* I'd ask myself. The grocery cart weighed a thousand pounds. I made myself speak to people, waited my turn in the check-out line, dreading the check-out girl's casual, "Hi. How are you?"

Since I love honesty, I learned to answer her question with something like, "Cold today, isn't it?" Sometimes I wanted to scream, "How do you think I am? My husband is staggering around the house with a brain tumor. How would you be?" But I managed never to do that. Getting groceries was one of the hard things. Chores that somehow brought a little relief were driving and folding clothes. . . .

The children, especially the boys, went about life pretty normally. Sometimes I was almost angry at their ability to laugh and go out and do fun things. Of course they believed with absolute certainty that their daddy was being healed. It was what he and I had taught them, and I wanted to believe it too. Oh, how I wanted to believe it.

Sometimes I could for brief periods of time. One of those times was when Jerry had a CAT scan done in January and the radiologist told us, "I see a shell where the tumor was."

The doctor was smiling from ear to ear. I made him repeat it five times. Rose, my friend from oncology, and another friend, Venera Weldon, were with us. I kept staring at the doctor. Venera grabbed me by the shoulders. "They can't find it, Marion!" Rose, who at one time had found emotional displays unattractive, began saying, "Thank You, Jesus! Praise You, Jesus!" at the top of her voice. They both threw their arms around Jerry and hugged him.

We all walked to the car with Rose repeating, "Thank You, Jesus!" I still had said nothing. Jerry was laughing out loud, Venera was crying and I walked along like a zombie. I got in under the steering wheel. Jerry climbed in the other side. Then it hit me like a tidal wave.

We have a second chance. We were going to grow old together. We could go downstairs and eat a bowl of cereal just the two of us after everyone was in bed. I could pick up his clothes at the cleaners. I could pick out greeting cards for him. He would pull up in the driveway at six, like always. His hair would grow back. We could see the boys graduate and be at Jennifer's wedding together. Oh, dear God, we were going to grow old together! *They couldn't find the tumor.* I bolted out of the car, screaming over my shoulder, "I have to tell Dr. Cunningham."

"Who?" Venera said.

"The cobalt doctor."

I ran like a crazy woman down the hall and nearly ran into Dr. Cunningham. "They can't find it!" I told him.

"What? What are you talking about?"

"The tumor. They can only find a shell."

"Of Jerry's tumor?" He didn't seem to believe me.

"Yes, go ask radiology. They've got a new CAT scan!"

"I've never heard of anything like this," he said.

"You've heard of prayer and miracles."

"Yes, of course."

"We've got one!" I called out over my shoulder as I ran back to the car.

We called people who'd been praying. The word spread like wildfire. Our phone nearly rang off the hook. The what-ifs didn't bother me that night. Jerry and I slept soundly, big C and little C, and the fear didn't move around inside me. I could feel faith, alive and strong. Until I was fully asleep, I kept whispering, *Thank You, Jesus.*

Then suddenly without warning a few weeks later, Jerry began acting strangely. He thought he saw more of things than were actually there and he decided Jennifer and I were plotting against him. He toyed with the clock continually, trying to figure out what time it was. I kept checking his eyes with a flashlight to see if they responded properly. I held up fingers and he couldn't tell me the correct number. We'd been warned that brain swelling could be as dangerous as the tumor and that it could progress very quickly once it began. I broke down and called Dr. Loren. I didn't want to. I wanted doctors out of our lives. I didn't even want to dial the number, but I did and she said what I expected, "Bring him to my office immediately."

I drove like an automaton refusing all emotions. Jerry cried all the way. We had just filled out forms to appear on *The 700 Club* to share Jerry's healing.

Dr. Loren said there was a large amount of swelling, but she changed his medication and didn't put him in the hospital. We drove home, grateful at least for this.

But the swelling continued. The next day Jerry accused Jennifer and me of scheming to put him in the hospital. He asked Jon and Jeremy if I were calling the doctor behind his back. Jennifer and I both told him over and over that we would do nothing without telling him, but the swelling was causing him to perceive things as they were not.

Finally, I got mad. He had been holding an alarm clock for

hours, talking about something being wrong with it. Then he'd gotten the calendar and tried to figure out what the date was. Something seemed to snap inside me and I permitted myself the luxury of anger. I hadn't done that throughout the entire illness. I grabbed the clock from him and slung it against the wall as hard as I could. It stunned both of us. It broke the clock, but it also seemed to break the tension. Jerry started to laugh, then I did too. Once again, his marvelous humor was rescuing us. I gave him extra swelling medicine and prayed a long time. I also got a prayer chain started.

The next morning things were more like normal—though a normal life now seemed little more than a fondly remembered dream. Oh, Lord, how good life had been once! Even our arguments over where to take a vacation seemed wonderful in retrospect. Jerry's reproaching me for picking up stray animals had been a game. Our problems with a rebellious teenager—Jennifer and I had gone through some difficult years—seemed routine now. When Julie got engaged at seventeen and I thought I'd die—that hadn't been so earth-shattering after all. The loneliness of living with someone who refused to express his thoughts would be child's play now.

Just five years ago there were six of us. Six plates on the table at meals. We took up six places in the pew at church, an entire booth in a restaurant. We filled up our car. Six people is a lot. Sometimes I had noticed people alone. That could never happen to me. I had the snug security of being surrounded by five people, even if we fussed sometimes. Sometimes I would look at our address labels and marvel over them: Mr. & Mrs. Jerry M. West. I adored being the other half of someone and seeing it in print. Sometimes when Jerry was silent and I didn't feel like a helpmeet, I'd pull out those labels and feel a warm, secure satisfaction. Loneliness was something far removed from me. Then suddenly Julie was gone. Married. Jennifer and her boyfriend, Charlie, were also talking about marriage "in a year or so." By then, Jerry would be dead. That would leave me with two boys—who'd always been closer to their father, anyway. And in a few years, the remorseless preview went on, they would be gone too and it would be . . . just me . . . alone. What would I do with this big house all alone?

I had to go to the grocery store late one afternoon about six. That scary time of day. Everywhere I looked there were only twosomes. What was this—couples' day? "Two by two they go marching through . . . Sweethearts on Parade. . . ." Pushing the shopping cart together, making selections together, standing in the check-out line together. Even the ones who were bickering looked wonderful to me. I watched a husband carrying groceries out to a car. Jerry used to have tremendous strength. There were so many things I didn't know how to do. I couldn't light the furnace. I didn't know about buying car tires or how to invest money. Who was the man who painted our house? I didn't understand expressways or North, South, East and West. I felt like a stranger in an even stranger land.

Like a top winding down Jerry moved slower and slower and everything was difficult for him. He stumbled a lot. "Please don't go to work tomorrow," I begged one night while I was helping him bathe.

"I'm going." For the first time I saw something in his eyes that frightened me. A new kind of fear welled up inside of me. It made me sick to my stomach as I identified it: I was afraid of Jerry! He was staring at me, not talking. I got him settled in bed, then sat down in a chair facing him.

You don't want to turn your back on him, I realized with horror. He'd never looked at me like this before. "You're going to take me to work," he repeated grimly.

"I won't." I spoke softly but my heart was pounding and my mouth was dry. If I called Dr. Loren and told her that there was a personality change, she would forbid him to go to work—I couldn't make myself do it. *I can't be afraid of gentle Jerry.* But he kept staring in that strange way. I went down to the living room and sat by the front door. How could this be happening?

After a while Jerry came down the steps—slowly, but managing by himself. I didn't move to help him. Tears filled his eyes. "Hiedy," he said.

I ran to him and we held onto each other. "Mannie, don't ever be afraid of me again."

The next morning he asked me in a quiet voice to take him to work.

"O.K., Jer." I didn't have strength anymore to argue or figure things out. Driving I prayed silently: *God, stop us some way if You know he shouldn't go to work. I'm all out of ideas. You have to do something.*

"Let's stop for lunch," Jerry said. Food was the furthest thing from my mind, but I'd do anything to delay this trip.

"Is Mary Mac's O.K.?" I asked. It was one of our favorite downtown restaurants.

"Yeah, that's fine."

I parked the car and we got out. He was moving incredibly slowly, looking around him as though we had landed on the moon. He didn't seem to know which way the restaurant was and waited for me to lead. I wouldn't. I stood still on the sidewalk while people went around us. *O God, help me do the right thing.* Jerry headed off in the wrong direction. I saw quick little seizures come and go.

"Let's go, love, back to the car."

"No! We're eating at Mary Mac's and then you're taking me to work."

"You don't know where you are."

"I'm just a little confused. Did I go the wrong way?"

"Please come with me, Jerry."

"I'm not going to let you ruin my career. You don't care. You're not thinking about me. Take me to work now." He was crying.

In the car I headed home while Jerry cried quietly. In the living room we sat and looked at each other. Finally, he said, "You don't know what it's like to put twenty-five years into a job and then just walk away. I can't give it up." He was still crying.

I thought, *I wish I could cry.* "I love you," I said and walked over and kissed him. "I'm going to call the office and tell them you aren't coming in."

"Tell them I'll be there tomorrow."

"No, Jer, I can't do that."

The people at Jerry's office seemed relieved that I had finally made a decision. Jerry continued to be devastated and if I could have experienced any emotions I'm sure I would have felt the devastation too, but I was fresh out of feelings. We sat in the living room and he cried softly with his face in his hands while I stared straight ahead. I was remembering a dance at Virginia Polytechnic Institute, where he went to college: Fats Domino singing, "I found my thrill on Blueberry Hill." I remembered the night he asked me to marry him. He wrote it on my back with his finger. I recalled those first married years. The babies arriving. The thrill of knowing we were expecting twins and how he looked when he learned he had two big boys. I remembered laughing with him. What fun we had laughing! Humor is one of the deepest emotions two people can share, a unique kind of love. I remembered the day we were broke and he brought me roses . . . for no special reason.

Then I remembered all those nights when he had to study for his professional engineer's license and I sat across the room crying and insisting that he didn't love me. I wrote him a love poem and he wouldn't stop studying to read it and I thought my heart would break. It took me a long time to realize that the romantic kind of love doesn't last through a marriage. He could have satisfied me in a second with a wink, a big smile, a quick kiss or almost any kind of comment, but he didn't know that, and I was terribly insecure.

Later I realized that something comes to replace romantic love. You really learn to love someone on days when you can't think of a thing you like about them, but you know you are committed to them . . . whatever. I thought Jerry was stubborn and selfish because he wouldn't stop studying and talk to me. But this new kind of love for him grew precisely because I couldn't control him. We must have been married fifteen years when it dawned on me that almost no one is really in love when he or she gets married. Newlyweds are "in" something. In infatuation. In agreement, in the mood, but not in love. They can't be in love when they only know the best about one another, only what the other wants them to know. I was amazed when I first discovered, "Why, you aren't what I thought you were . . . but I think I'm going to love you anyway." I'm sure he felt the same way about me. I would have enjoyed talking with him about it, but he didn't like such conversations.

I was spoiled at the time we were married. I didn't even know how to shop for groceries. I slept till noon, hated cooking and wanted to pick up every stray animal I saw. During the first weeks of marriage I threw away five bell peppers. Jerry saw them in the trash can and asked, "Why did you throw them out?"

"They were all hollow," I replied.

He just looked at me for a long time.

I wasn't frugal. Our temperaments were entirely different. His life seemed to center around food and sports and work. I thought maybe someday he'd write me a love note and leave it on the pillow. One morning during the first year of marriage, I did find a note on the refrigerator. It said, "Something in here stinks. Clean it out!"

When he ignored me too long, I could usually entice him into an argument. Anything was better than silence. I remembered a familiar area of disagreement. Time. Jerry loved to be late, while I always wanted to be the first one anywhere. One evening I threw his clothes in the tub with him because he wouldn't hurry. He methodically wrung them out and of course that night we were even later. I remembered too that Jerry said something funny and got us laughing over it. After Julie was married, she said, "Know what I miss the most about being away from home? Hearing y'all laugh. It used to give me the best feeling." She never mentioned the arguments.

Recently Jerry had fallen in the bathroom and I couldn't get him up. He pulled me down with him and we just lay there, laughing.

So many thoughts crowded my mind as I sat looking at him. "Twenty-five years is a long time, Marion. I love my job."

"I know. You're good at it, too. And the people there love you."

He buried his face in his hands and said, "Oh, God, this is hard."

I looked out the window at the cars. Men were coming home from work. Some of them would fight with their wives. Maybe some wouldn't even speak. Some would embrace at the door. Whatever they were facing, I envied them at that moment.

"You want something to eat, Jer?"

"No, babe, I can't eat." He'd just started calling me that after all these years. I loved it. I stood up and looked at him.

"How did you manage to get such a dud to marry?" he said.

"Take it back," I warned.

"O.K., O.K."

I went over to him and we held onto each other without talking. I no longer bugged him to talk to me. He loved me. He really loved me. Why had it taken us so long to learn to love one another unconditionally?

8

The Little Gray Man

There was no schedule in our days now. Radiation was finished; Jerry had stopped working. The days were endless, except when loyal friends came by with food, prayers and hope. Jerry greeted them eagerly: He could never get enough of talking about Jesus. The sports page was now a forgotten thing, often never even unfolded. Sometimes he wanted me to read his Bible to him. His eyesight wasn't so good, even though he'd just gotten new glasses.

One day we were alone as the long afternoon closed in on us, like a creeping enemy. We sat propped up in bed because Jerry felt better lying down and I wanted to be close to him. We listened to the ticking of the clock. *God*, I prayed, *do something. Send someone.*

Sure enough, in a little while the doorbell rang. I practically flew down the steps and opened the door. An enormous stranger stood there. He had piercing blue eyes and carried a Bible in his hand. "Hi, I'm George Smith—starting a new fellowship in this area. I have an appointment somewhere else, but . . . my car just turned in here. Do you folks have a church? Is there any way I could help you?"

"Yes, George, we have a church, but we also have a need right now!" I decided not to beat around the bush. "Satan is devouring us," I told this heaven-sent stranger. "My husband has brain cancer. We've had some victories, but we're in deep defeat now. Not only in his body, but in our spirits. Don't come in unless you mean business and want to get in the battle with us. Don't come in just to be polite."

George nearly knocked me over. "Which way?" He looked like an enormous tackle on a winning football team. Somehow I felt George Smith was already a friend. I knew that Jerry would like him too.

"Up the steps."

He ran up ahead of me, taking them three at a time. "Hello, brother," he greeted Jerry and bent over to hug him. They embraced for a long time. Then George fell to his knees, laid his hands on Jerry's shoulders and began to pray. I looked at Jerry's eyes. They were closed, but the radiance, the glow was back. He looked victorious again. After the prayer we sat around and talked for a long time. George became a regular visitor and always seemed to come when we needed him most.

It had stopped surprising me. From the beginning of our ordeal, whenever the battle was fiercest, God had sent help. I remembered the time, in Intensive Care, before we knew what Jerry's problem was, when my faith had hit rock bottom. With my head against the cold metal rail of Jerry's bed, I had prayed, *God, send someone to encourage us.*

At that moment I heard a booming voice. It sounded like Charlton Heston in a Bible movie: "I am the Lord God who strengthens you. Yea, with My mighty right hand I will uphold you. Fear not. . . ."

I bolted out into the hall and traced the magnificent voice to another Intensive Care cubicle. A tall, erect, young black man stood reading the Bible to the frail-looking woman in the bed. He glanced at me. "We need you, next door," I whispered.

He smiled and nodded.

In a few minutes he appeared by Jerry's bed. Jerry had been sleeping, but it wasn't a good, natural sleep. He opened his eyes

as the tall stranger began reading the ninety-first Psalm, one of
our favorites.

"Could you sing?" I pleaded.

"I don't sing," he laughed.

"But could you sing anyway?"

He took a deep breath and began, "Blessed assurance, Jesus is
mine. . . ."

Jerry was smiling. So was I. Our faith was soaring again. We
joined in singing with the young man, then held hands and prayed.

"Who are you?" I finally asked.

"I'm a believer," he smiled.

"Do you have a name, Believer?"

"Jerry Hutchins." Somehow I felt it was an added bond that
he and my Jerry should have the same name. "I work for an
insurance company," he went on. "I come here nights to pray
for my aunt and I preach on the weekends. It's the first time I've
ever sung, though."

"I think you're going to be singing a lot, Jerry."

He hugged us both and promised to return the next night. Even
after my Jerry went home, he'd come to visit and sing for us.

Was it this succession of supportive presences—provided so
regularly by God—that made possible what happened next? I
can't be sure. I only know that one day a miraculous healing did
occur . . . in me.

I woke up one morning feeling as if an elephant were sitting on
my chest. The silent voices were chanting, *Your husband's dying*. . . . As desperate as Jerry's situation was, I felt desperate
too. How could I help and support him, when there was no
energy or faith left in me?

I started crying. It was the second time during the whole crisis
that tears had come. "Help me," I finally asked. "Something is
devouring me on the inside."

Jerry grabbed the Bible and began to read and pray for me. For
a while we put his problems to one side in order to concentrate on
mine. "Marion," Jerry said suddenly, "there is a word from
your childhood that you need to say . . . a word you don't want

to say. Just one word. Think. What is it? God wants to heal you of something.''

I knew right away what the word was. I could see it in my mind in big fat letters. "Yes," I almost screamed.

"Say it," Jerry commanded.

"No."

"You have to, to get help."

"I can't."

He prayed over me, putting his hands on my head as I went through a fierce inner struggle. The phone rang and Jerry briefly explained the situation to the caller who promised to join in praying. "Marion, say the word!" Jerry grabbed me by the shoulders, almost roughly.

"No."

Daddy. I could see the word on the greeting card. I'd found it when I was a little girl. Even then I couldn't say it. I kept the card for years and looked at it often, but I wouldn't say the word.

Jerry was crying now. "You have to, Mannie, in the name of Jesus. You have to be free. I need you free of fear."

The word was in my mouth and Jerry was waiting.

I opened my mouth and whispered as softly as possible, "Daddy."

"You never knew him, did you?"

I shook my head, unable to say any more.

"Say it again."

"Daddy."

"He loved you."

"He left me."

I could see the greeting card now. A little girl sitting up in her father's lap with his arms around her. The printed message read, "Happy Father's Day to my Daddy." The man and the little girl were wearing clothes from the late 1930s. I would have been one or two when my mother picked it out. On the inside she'd signed it for me: "Love, Marion."

We got up and got dressed. All during the morning I said the word again. "Daddy." And gradually, amazingly, I discovered

I was saying it without fear or resentment or feelings of rejection. I told Jerry about the card, told him how I used to get it out and play with it and pretend that my father was still alive. I remembered that when I played paper dolls with my friends, I'd pretend that their fathers were dead and mine was alive.

Something was healing inside me—perhaps because God had shown us that we weren't abandoned, whatever the appearance. That He could send even total strangers to fill the gaps in our lives. That afternoon, Dru Glisson and Caryl Swift came over and had a long prayer session with me. Someone had taken Jerry to Jon's basketball game. Dru and Caryl and I ended up kneeling on the floor of the recreation room. Things that had been inside me a long time began coming out. Fear came out first. I got a vivid, unforgettable mental picture of the fear leaving. It was a stooped little man, all gray, with a gray ragged coat that dragged behind him and a floppy gray hat. His clothes and skin were all the same color. He was looking back over his shoulder with resentment, angry because he was being made to leave in the name of Jesus. Other things went too, but mostly I remember that picture and how I knew immediately that his name was fear and that he'd been in me a very long time. I didn't understand what was happening but I knew it was something God had been waiting for. He gave my two friends special power and discernment to help me that day.

When it was over I stood up and took a deep breath. I'll never forget the sensation. It was as though a breath mint had gone deep into my soul and everything was clean and fresh and pure all the way through me, down to my toes.

I went to the basketball game and joined Jerry. I talked to the people in the bleachers around us, and laughed. I thought, *I'm back in the real world again.* God was very close, even at the ball game. I thought I heard Him say, *You were a long time in dealing with that. I'm pleased with you.*

I cheered at the game with Jerry when Jon scored and I didn't resent couples there without a problem like ours. Oh, it was so good not to resent. I kept talking to people and laughing.

The next morning the most amazing thing happened. I woke up before Jerry, like always. But . . . something was different. What was it? I listened, not knowing what I was listening for.

Silence.

O God, beautiful silence! The voices, the chanting, menacing voices that had screamed at me each morning *were gone*.

"Thank You, Jesus! I don't understand what happened or even what it was called, but thank You. I don't think I could have stood them another day."

9

The Re-creation Room

Fear of course tried to come back in, and I had to resist. My mind was clear enough now to read the Bible. I went over and over the Scriptures on fear, confirming that it is definitely not God's will for His children to be afraid. I was aware that the mean little gray man named fear would try any way in the world to come back into my life again. He was nearby, just waiting for his chance.

Meanwhile Jerry and I grew closer and closer. Only a few years before he had told me, "We don't have anything in common anymore. You've changed." He was afraid of my obsession with Jesus. Had I been smarter I would not have kept insisting there is "something more." The more I nagged, the further away he moved.

But now I was living with a new man . . . a new creation in the same old earth suit, filled with power and joy. We had set up hospital facilities in the recreation room. We hadn't moved Jerry there, but everything was ready should he eventually not be able to go up and down steps to our bedroom. I liked to call it a re-creation room because I felt strongly that a great miracle would occur there.

Jerry had so many headaches now. We put hot cloths on him constantly—once I even blistered his head with them. He didn't

72

complain about the blisters or about the headaches. He rubbed his head until he rubbed off some skin, but he would not complain. How I admired him!

I searched constantly for new cancer treatments. I heard about one drug manufactured in a distant state. The F.D.A. had given the chemist who'd come up with the formula a patent number, so I wasn't dealing with a quack. Only cancer patients with no hope were allowed to try the medicine. We qualified, and I got some of the promising drug shipped to us.

There were various clinics, too, all claiming astonishing cures. Two in particular, neither of them in this country, I wanted Jerry to try. He refused. "We're not going through that. God can work here as well as anywhere. I don't want to leave our home and our friends." It wouldn't have made much difference if we had gone. I know that now. I obtained Jerry's medical records when I began this book. On January 4, 1983, Dr. Loren had written: "I think Mr. West realizes the seriousness of his diagnosis and realizes that there is a great possibility of a progressive downhill in the future. The patient's wife is calling all over the country to various medical centers and she has given me a list of names she wants me to check out . . . she is, of course, desperate."

That desperation, had I but known it, is the final step before one can enter into Nevertheless Living. . . .

Although Jerry refused to go dashing about the world in search of cures, he was more than willing to try any treatment available locally. Medical opinion was divided as to whether chemotherapy would do any good. One doctor frankly advised against it: "It's an ordeal to go through. I wouldn't take it if it were me." But Jerry was insistent that he be on some kind of a program. It was unthinkable to him not to have a plan. "They say it will make you sick," I told him.

"I'll be fine," he insisted. "I want to take it."

It did not require being hospitalized: The injections could be given in the doctor's office, and some of the medicine I could give him at home.

I found my solace once again in sorting clothes and doing the laundry. It was simple and familiar. White things, colored things and towels. It was a sweetly familiar routine in stark contrast to reading the directions for the chemotherapy medications and coping with the dreaded side effects. I liked to take the clothes warm from the dryer and put my face in them . . . hide in the warmth for a moment. The fear was trying to come back.

The day we went for the first chemotherapy injection, Jerry laughed and joked and helped the nurse feel comfortable. He didn't complain when he threw up the next day. I kept working at refusing fear. It was an exhausting task and I wasn't always successful.

It was about two weeks later that Jerry began to have difficulty in both walking and speaking. Our practical nurse friend Rose came over and despite her cheerful manner, I sensed deep concern. I was so grateful she had come. When you are desperate and alone it is marvelous to see someone drive up who will help you make decisions. Rose suggested it was time to move Jerry into the re-creation room. She went out and got all the things that a real hospital room would have. A portable toilet, an eating tray, a walker, a wheelchair, notebooks for nurses. She even arranged for a telephone; her husband, Glenn, came over and connected it for us. The Cancer Society of our county supplied everything we needed, free of cost.

I recalled the time, two years previously, when Rose told me she had volunteered to work on the oncology floor at the hospital. I had wondered: Why would anyone want to work with cancer patients? Rose began coming over daily for a six-hour shift.

The re-creation room was large and cheerful, with red carpeting and a sleep sofa. There were family pictures on the walls, along with football and basketball trophies. The stereo was there so we kept praise music going all the time. Our favorite tape was: "Communion: A Sing-A-Long for God's People in Harmony." An address label I'd stuck on the cassette said: Mr. & Mrs. Jerry M. West."

10

The Island

One evening as Jerry was undressing to go to bed, down in the re-creation room, he toppled over backwards. He felt stiff like a store mannequin. His eyes were open and there were no spasms or jerking, just unbelievable stillness. I hadn't seen a seizure like this before. He didn't seem to be breathing and for a moment I thought he was dead.

Then he moved a little, but a few minutes later, after Jon and Jeremy and Jennifer had helped me get him onto the bed, another seizure hit. We couldn't make any contact with him, although his eyes were open. The ambulance came and Dr. Loren met us at the now familiar emergency room. *O God, I can't fill out the forms again, answer the questions. A hospital is where you go to get well. They can't help him. Why are we here?* Julie had met us there and seemed to know what I was thinking. "Go on with Daddy, Mother, I can answer the questions."

Dr. Loren found enormous brain swelling, the thing we had so dreaded. "Actually, Marion, since I've gone over the CAT scans, I don't know how he ever went back to work. It was physically impossible. He's the most remarkable man I've ever known. I love him. He's made a tremendous impact on me. I want you to know this is very, very serious. I don't think you realize how serious."

I realized, all right. Only, I was working so hard at not giving in to fear that I wasn't allowing any emotions inside at all.

"If he stops breathing," Dr. Loren went on, "do you want him put on a respirator? I have to put it on his chart." I stared at her in silence. More decisions. "I'll talk to the children." I said.

We sat on the floor in the hallway and discussed it. Julie jumped up and said, "Of course we want him on the respirator! I'll go tell her." I stared at the yellow wall and people's feet as they walked by us. It was past midnight. I didn't really think that decision would come up tonight or anytime soon; I believed Dr. Loren just wanted to be certain I understood that Jerry might die. Julie came back and sat down. "How are we going to get through this night?" I asked.

"Five minutes at a time," Julie said. "We can do anything five minutes at a time."

At Dr. Loren's suggestion we rented a room in the hospital where we took turns lying down. From time to time one of the children went down to I.C.U. to check on Jerry. Finally it was morning. Jerry was stable for the time being, sleeping soundly. We went home to change clothes.

For the next three days I drove back and forth between the house and the hospital. And it was on one of these trips, on a spring evening, May 11, 1983, that God did something in my life that I have great difficulty understanding, let alone explaining. The greatest change—the greatest miracle—of my life occurred. Nevertheless Living began.

The brain swelling had gone down some and Jerry was to go home the next day, although we knew a recurrence could happen at any time. I was driving home alone from the hospital early in the evening. The sun was setting. I hated sunsets. They used to be romantic, but no longer. *I'm alone*, I thought.

"You know I didn't want to be alone, God. You knew that." We were back on good terms, and I could speak to Him as always. He had been very patient with me, waiting until I was ready to talk.

Suddenly it seemed as though the sun's rays came right inside the car. Everything around me appeared golden. I felt golden, too. And . . . not at all alone. Something very close to peace and joy seemed to have come into the car with me. For a moment I wondered if the car was going to just float up off the highway. It wasn't scary. It was golden and beautiful. That's the only way I can describe it. *Something good is about to happen,* I thought. It had been so long since I'd experienced anything good. After a few minutes the gold feeling left the car, but not the sense of expectation.

At home things were in utter confusion. We were getting new carpet. It seemed ridiculous, but Jerry had wanted it. He had picked out the color, Canyon Clay . . . a lovely shade of brown. All the furniture was piled up and I had to climb over things to get to our bedroom. I did it without thinking twice. I had been climbing over things mentally and emotionally for months. I could surely climb over a little furniture. But the enemy jumped in and insisted, *See how confusing everything is? This is how it's going to be for the rest of your life. Things will never be normal again. Why don't you just give up? Your life is over. Go around that curve and end it all. Go fast around that curve.*

But I kept remembering the golden experience and the hint of peace and joy I had just felt on the highway. Suppose that could happen again? Suppose it could be a lifestyle, regardless of what life dished out? *How silly to get new carpet,* the enemy mocked, *when you don't have a husband.*

But God was talking about the carpet, too. *You are going to be walking in new areas, child. It's good to start out by walking on new carpet. It represents new places in your life where you'll be venturing. I want you to have it. Rejoice.*

Of course the enemy tried to tell me that God didn't care about carpets, of all things, and that it was only my imagination. But I knew God was telling me something. In response to Him while I got dressed to go back to the hospital I sang a little song. One I hadn't sung in a long time, and one I didn't feel like singing then: "This is the day, this is the day that the Lord hath made! I will rejoice, I will rejoice, and be glad in it!"

I had a good visit with Jerry that evening; he was coming home the next day at noon. *Maybe,* I thought, *the wonderful thing will happen then.* But it happened, in fact, before that; it happened at dawn, just as I was waking. I wasn't the least bit drowsy, and there was a question formed and waiting on my mind: *Father, where am I in my spiritual walk now? What's happening?*

I could imagine God smiling and saying, *I'm glad you asked that.* He seemed to go on to explain: *You are at the crucial moment now. You have been shipwrecked and nearly drowned in icy waters of fear. But you've kept swimming and you are within reach of an island. Right now you can crawl up on the shore and be safe there.*

"Father, what is the name of the island?"

It's called the Island of Trust. You will be alone on it, but you will be safe. If you stay on it, nothing will hurt you.

I imagined myself crawling up on the island. I was getting out of the cold, choppy waters. The white sand on the island was warm, like clothes out of the dryer. I lay down on the sand. There were palm trees and a flag on the island. The flag was red with white letters and they spelled "Trust." It flapped in the wind.

"I want to stay here, God."

I want you here. You need to know that all kinds of well-meaning people will come to try to rescue you. They'll come in boats of various kinds, and encourage you to swim out to them. You might be tempted to walk out just a little way. You must not even put your feet in the water. You will experience fear again if you get off the Island of Trust. The water is dangerous. This is the only place of safety for you. I'm so happy that you finally got here, child.

"Me, too. It feels so good here. I don't want to swim and struggle in those dark waters anymore. I think I want to be a vessel, after all. I want to be available to You. I'd like to help other fearful people get to this island. I know it's a real place. I want to give myself to You in a new way . . . and I want to give Jerry to you, too. . . ."

Of course, child. I received him with great love. He was never yours, anyway. Nor are you yours. You gave yourself to Me a long time ago. I know how to care for Jerry. Doesn't it feel good to have given up the struggle? It's all my struggle now. You could have done this long ago. But I understand you and how your mind and emotions have to struggle. Relinquishment is very hard. Many people find it impossible, so they never reach this wonderful island that I have prepared for My shipwrecked children.

Then God gave me a Scripture: "We are more than conquerors through him [Christ Jesus] who loved us." In the early morning light, I found it in the eighth chapter of Romans, verse 37. Funny, I never knew it said *more* than conquerors. I thought it just said, conquerors.

"What's the 'more,' Lord?"

No words came to me. Just a clear mental picture. It was of a ladder. On each rung was a word: warrior, soldier, conqueror and other words that I couldn't see. The ladder went up very high into the clouds. The top rung was above the clouds and on that rung was written *More than a conqueror. Jerry is going to be more than a conqueror. You'll see. Stay on the island. Don't leave it! You couldn't have even looked at the ladder without fear if you hadn't been on the Island of Trust.*

"I trust You, Father." I must have said it fifty times. I understood the picture. Jerry would be healed . . . with Jesus. Not here on earth as we had all prayed. I still believed that God healed physical bodies. I just knew that Jerry would be healed in another dimension, and that incredibly . . . it was all right. The Island of Trust is a remarkable place indeed.

My struggle had come to an end. I didn't have to hold on anymore. I'd been holding on for so long. I didn't have to try to control anything. I could rest at last on this sweet, marvelous island. Do nothing except to trust. God was in control. It wasn't my battle. Praise God! The battle was the Lord's. Tears of joy stung my eyes. I sat up on my knees and looked out the window. The sunrise didn't frighten me at all. Birds sang in the old oak tree. I didn't resent their song anymore. "Thank you," I whispered. I was excited about my victory and Jerry's too. I didn't understand it, but I knew that God was going to give us both a victory.

You're crazy. You've finally flipped under the pressure, the enemy blustered.

He couldn't touch me on the island. I knew it. He did, too.

That, so far as I can recall, was the first time I used the actual word "nevertheless" in this kind of situation, though of course I hadn't even begun yet to grasp all that it implied. I told the enemy out loud, "Nevertheless, Satan, you might take notice that I'm not afraid. That's joy in my heart. Joy! The fear is gone."

There was no response.

I hummed while I dressed. What a God! He seemed to show me another mental picture. It was quick . . . just a glimpse. A purple velvet curtain with a gold cord moved back for a brief instant and I saw myself in some new kind of life . . . a ministry of some sort.

Words came to my mind easily. *You have another life to live. I am in control. There's something you have to do. You are a chosen vessel. I have chosen you very carefully. You can't understand now. It's too soon. Just trust. Every breath you take, trust Me. No matter what happens. You are going to be fine. Your days of fear are finally over. You've been afraid all your life. It's possible to live fear-free, Marion.*

I drove down the highway to bring Jerry home singing "Praise the Name of Jesus. . . ." Entering the hospital I smiled and spoke to people. I walked tall and straight. It was a beautiful morning. I didn't have to figure out anything or struggle anymore. I saw myself standing on the Island of Trust. I'd never known such intense love as I found on the island. As I rode up in the elevator the words of a psalm came to my mind:

"He sent from above, he took me, he drew me out of many waters."

11

The Vessel

The enemy obviously didn't like what was happening. It would be midday before Jerry was discharged. We chatted for a while in his hospital room. Then, as Jerry drifted off to sleep, Satan jumped in with a negative thought. He reminded me of a dream I had had from time to time for the past ten years or so. I have always had very vivid dreams, frequently in color; I can still recall dreams from my childhood.

In the recurring dream, we were living happily in Atlanta. Then suddenly deep fear would come over me; the sun would go behind a cloud and it would be dark and cold. A voice in the dream would insist, *There's no one for you. You are alone. No one loves you. You don't have a "someone" like other women.* And that feeling I had known as a child when other little girls held their daddies' hands would return.

Yes, I do have someone, I would shout back. *I have Jerry. We've been married for years. This is just a dream. I'll always have him. I'll show you.* Then in the dream I would begin to look around for Jerry in all the familiar places, while all the time it grew darker and colder. I could never find him. *Jerry!* I would scream.

Finally I would force myself awake and reach for Jerry in the bed. "Whatsamatter?" he would mumble, still asleep.

"Make a big C," I'd beg. He would curl around me and I would feel safe . . . until the dream came again.

Watching Jerry sleeping in the hospital bed now, I decided that victory must first be mental. I knew I had been slow in learning that truth. I decided to combat the negative images of the dream with every positive recent memory I could muster. Just last month, April 12th had been our twenty-fifth anniversary. Jerry had sent a dozen red roses with a card that said, "Thank you for twenty-five wonderful years. I love you." He had still been working half-days then and I rushed to the phone to call him. He had laughed and for a few moments it was like old times.

The children and my mother had planned an anniversary treat for us, an overnight stay at Stone Mountain Inn, a world-famous resort just five minutes from our home. They had reserved the honeymoon suite for us, with a canopied four poster bed. Julie had insisted that I take along the matching gown and robe she'd worn on her honeymoon.

The next morning the boys had a baseball game. It was unseasonably cold, but Jerry wanted to go. He watched them play intently, howling encouragement. I no longer resented his enthusiasm. It was so good to have a husband to sit by at a ballgame, even if I didn't understand the action.

Jerry woke up and I helped him get out of bed and into his clothes. We were going home. Somehow I knew he would not have to come back to the hospital again. . . .

At home I got him settled on the sofa, fixed him something to drink and gave him a round of medicine. I wanted him to eat, but he was losing his appetite. As I unpacked his suitcase, I remembered the comic books I had collected as a child. There was a certain ad in all of them. The picture showed a "90-pound weakling" sitting helplessly on the beach while a big bully kicked sand in his face. Determined to defend himself, the skinny young man developed the "Charles Atlas Body-Building" course. In just a few short weeks he became the muscle man of the beach and walked wherever he wanted in total victory.

Somehow I had discovered the spiritual equivalent of the

Charles Atlas course. I wasn't certain of its name yet, but I knew it existed.

I had discovered the reality of "They that wait upon the Lord shall renew their strength; they shall mount up with wings as eagles; they shall run, and not be weary; and they shall walk and not faint." I added a passage: "They shall care for their husbands with joy and without fear—no matter what. They shall leave fear behind as surely as a snake leaves his old skin and moves on."

Still marveling over my discovery, I asked, "God, could You give me another mental picture? They help me so much. I have surrendered Jerry to You. You are his loving Father. I will not give him over to the enemy. Give me a picture that I can hold onto when Satan tries to tell me he has won."

I waited. Then in my mind I saw a group of children eating ice cream cones. One little boy—it was obviously Jerry—didn't have one. He was watching the other children so wistfully. I wanted to cry out, "He's missing something!" I didn't want Jerry to miss out on *anything*—seeing the boys graduate from high school, giving Jennifer away when she married, watching Jamie grow up, getting to know other grandchildren still to be born. . . . "O Father, he's going to miss those things! The enemy can remind me of that!"

God interrupted my panicky thoughts: *Marion, that little boy with no ice cream cone holds the franchise to all the Baskin Robbins stores in the nation in his hip pocket. Trust Me.*

"O Father, he isn't really going to miss anything, is he? You are going to show him great and mighty things that I can't imagine. I do trust You."

The next day while I was vacuuming, God gave me another picture. I saw a car rolling down a hill, out of control. Jerry was in it, but the brakes had failed. The car was heading for a high cliff. I wanted to scream, "Jump, Jerry, jump!" and then, right at the brink of the cliff, a loving hand reached in and pulled Jerry to safety and only the empty car went over. *Jerry's going to be all right, Marion, I promise you. You are, too. All the hard part is over, now that you are on the Island of Trust.*

"I want to tell You, Father," I responded, "that I fully realize no one is taking him from me. I give him to You. I let go. It almost feels like . . . worship. It's not my battle."

It never was, but I had to let you wear yourself out and come to Me beaten and all out of ideas before I could hold you and reassure you. You held on for so long. Many dear children never let go. They hold on for a lifetime, even after someone is gone. This earthly existence is like a play. Each one is assigned a part, with the proper entrances and exits. You are just in the play. For a long time you were trying to direct it.

"You're so much bigger that I knew. Who would ever have thought that I could let go and have all this joy, too?"

I remembered once burning my hand very badly. The only relief I found was to stand at the faucet and let cold water stream over it. Now Jesus, the Living Water, was giving me relief and I couldn't bear to move away. My mind and spirit and body were all standing in the stream. Never mind the circumstances. God was not limited by circumstances.

He is the God of Nevertheless. It was the first time the sentence had come to me. *God is not a God of what-if; He is the God of Nevertheless.*

"Whatever You choose is fine with me, Father," I went on. "I'm not trying to direct the play anymore. I am fully convinced that You are bringing about something marvelous and that Jerry and I will both continue to live in victory, even if we aren't together. I don't understand this, but I do believe. No one will understand my joy, but I don't care. It's real."

Don't talk about it yet. Just ponder it for a while. The time will come when you can share it. Now is not the time. I am going to use all of this. Nothing will be wasted. Trust Me. I have something for you to do. No one else can do it. Don't indulge in any self-pity whatsoever or I cannot use you.

"I won't, Father. Use me any way You want to. I long to be a vessel. I'm excited about being a vessel." I remembered the day at the luncheon when I told God I would not be a vessel. Now I had changed my mind. If I were not to be a vessel, I would have no reason to live. I almost laughed aloud. "O Father, I hope it's not in the church nursery or in the kitchen!"

I think He laughed, too. We both remembered all the years I had volunteered for the nursery because I wanted to look good and no one else would do it. How I hated it! "Let me reach hurting, fearful people. Oh, I want to do that. Give me a ministry to fearful people. I understand the terrible clutches of fear and how life isn't worth living if you have to live it in fear. Empower me to help other people.

"Oops, Father, I'm getting ahead of You, aren't I? I'm so bad about that. But I'll learn."

I began dressing carefully, taking time to put on makeup and match my clothes. I did it to erase the memories of all those days I sat in my robe and stared ahead, frozen in fear, so close to a breakdown. The enemy had convinced me my life and certainly my joy was over. He had me believing I would live like a zombie—if I chose to continue living.

And in that condition of total defeat, when I had no will to go on fighting, I had somehow stumbled into Nevertheless Living. The words of Isaiah 61 had literally come true: God had given *me* "beauty for ashes, the oil of joy for mourning, the garment of praise for the spirit of heaviness."

The garment of praise. I decided I would go out and buy some new clothes to take care of Jerry in. I wanted to look pretty for him. I knew, oh, I knew that we were *both* going to be more than conquerors. I didn't know how. But it wasn't my problem.

I decided I could finish my *Guideposts* devotionals after all, and sat down and wrote the other fifteen that were due in one sitting. It didn't seem possible that the typewriter was going clickety-click again. I loved the sound of it and the touch of it. My mind was functioning in a creative way. Maybe someday I would write another book after all.

12

The Inward Man

The chemotherapy continued to affect Jerry's appetite. He ate little and lost much of that. The headaches continued. Rose came regularly for a five- or six-hour shift, usually during the night so I could sleep. We had everything we needed in the re-creation room and God repeatedly assured me that Jerry would not go back to the hospital. I was so grateful for that knowledge. Jerry still radiated the love of Jesus. He couldn't seem to stop smiling and I was soaring . . . fear-free. I knew positively that I could care for him here.

A doctor phoned to suggest that I might want to see a counselor so that I could better face what lay ahead. "Finances, for example," he said. "Have you had experience handling money?"

"Not much," I answered truthfully. Anything about numbers confused me, and I'd given up years ago trying to understand bank statements or income tax forms.

The doctor continued, "You simply are not prepared for what is about to happen. A counselor can help you face reality."

"I am prepared, doctor, and I'm fine."

"You can't be fine facing what you are facing."

"But I am fine. And I have a counselor. Wait—I'll give you the Scripture." I grabbed my Bible. " 'When my heart was embittered and I was pierced within . . . Nevertheless, I am continually with thee, thou hast taken hold of my right hand. With thy counsel thou wilt guide me.' That's in Psalm 73. And here—here's another one. 'I will bless the Lord who counsels me.' That's Psalm 16.''

Eventually and politely, with a sort of I-warned-you tone in his voice, the doctor said goodbye. He was a dear man. He just didn't understand about nevertheless.

Jerry could get out of the hospital bed with help, but it was very difficult. He could not make his limbs do what he wanted them to do. I got him up one day by myself and into the wheelchair and took him out back. Caleb, our collie, seemed to understand that they wouldn't romp today and sat quietly by the wheelchair.

In the chair I could see the great change in Jerry's physical condition. His body was like those concentration camp photos: gaunt, emaciated. We sat on the patio in the afternoon sun. It was the middle of June. Usually we'd be planning a vacation at this time of year.

Back in the re-creation room, as Jeremy and I were helping him out of the chair, Jerry fell. The two of us went down with him and all three of us lay in a heap, laughing. "Jeremy, go across the street and get Mike." Mike was a young neighbor who often helped out. Jeremy didn't move. "Jeremy, go on, son."

"I can't. Daddy's lying on my foot." We all laughed harder and I tugged at Jeremy's foot until it was free. He sprinted out the door and was back in a flash with Mike, who picked Jerry up and got him back into bed. I knew I couldn't get Jerry up anymore. I think he knew it too, but we didn't mention it. I crawled up in the hospital bed with him and asked, "Who's the President, Jer?"

It's a question neurologists love. Jerry didn't know who the President was. I knew he didn't know. "It's not Nixon, is it?"

"No," I said.

Then a marvelous smile crossed his face and I knew he'd come up with something better than the right answer.

"I am," he teased.

I threw my head back and laughed. "Then I'm the First Lady."

He kissed me and held me close. The cat jumped up in the bed with us and I thanked God silently that we could be at home. We looked out of the window at the front yard . . . enormous trees that Jerry had planted when we first moved into the house twelve years ago, lawnmowers hummed, children ran by the window, cars zoomed past in the street.

People continued to come and pray with us, bringing so much food that I didn't cook for three months. Jerry always ended up praying for the needs of the people who came, rather than his own. As his body and even his mind deteriorated his love for God and for other people grew to enormous proportions.

One day Julie came by with Jamie who was now a year and a half. "Hey, Grady," she said—her name for Jerry.

Julie picked her up and placed her on Jerry's bed and he gave her a big hug. Then he opened his arms for Julie. "Come here, honey." She dropped down into his arms and they embraced for ever so long. I'd never known him to hold any of the children like that. Learning to express love had been a long time in coming to Jerry and he was making up for lost time with all of us. She told me almost a year later that that embrace was one of the dearest moments of her life. "I'd wanted him to hold me for so long."

One day Jerry told the boys, "Don't ever be ashamed of Jesus. He's the most important thing in your life. Don't push Him over in a corner and just be religious. Make Him number one."

"Yes, sir," they both said together. For eleven years I had prayed to hear Jerry say that to our sons. A mother can say it day after day, but a boy needs to hear that from his father. I used to hear Jerry tell the twins about certain sports figures, wishing he'd talk to them with the same enthusiasm about Jesus.

The boys never questioned me about Jerry's condition. Obviously he was failing fast, but I didn't want to butt in where the Holy Spirit might be explaining things to them. When Jon found a passage in 2 Corinthians to fit the situation, I knew I'd made the right decision. "Hey, Mama, this is what's happening to Daddy.

Listen. 'For which cause we faint not; but though our outward man perish, yet the inward man is renewed day by day.' ''

He understood, and I suspected Jeremy and the girls did too. At last I was learning to keep quiet.

13

The Train Ride

Because on my island there was no fear whatsoever, I was able to get the clothes ready for Jerry's homegoing—just as I had when he was going off on a business trip. It didn't really matter what he wore, because I knew he was dressed in the righteousness of Christ, but he was always picky about clothes. I chose a suit I had bought for his birthday—very expensive and not on sale. Julie had been with me and had seen me looking at it. "Oh, Mother, get it for him!"

The next instructions I got from my Father were to let the children make the selection of a coffin. I don't like the word, but there's nothing else to call it. The four of them stood quietly and listened to my instructions. "Jon, you know about wood," I said, "so you have the final say. I don't want anything shiny. Maybe oak, very simple. You'll know when you see it."

He nodded. "I can handle it, Mom." He was taking woodworking in school and was hurrying with his first project, a telephone table, so Jerry could see it. He has a real way with his hands, like Jerry's dad.

One of our best friends, a man who attended Bible studies at our house, worked at the funeral home, where they made the selection. It meant a great deal to me to know Bob Frahm was helping them. I knew he would understand our victory. God was certainly supplying our needs according to His riches in Christ Jesus, just as He promised.

When they got back, Jon said, "Mama, I hope it's all right, but I sort of . . . enjoyed doing that. I knew it the minute I saw it. I mean it's so nice and . . . it looks like Daddy. I almost wish he could see it. I made the right selection, Mama. It was like someone showing me which one to get."

"Thanks, Jon."

"I wanted to do it. Thank you for letting us go by ourselves."

Jerry's condition worsened and Rose brought in another nurse, Jean Thomas. Jean also worked on the oncology floor at the hospital and knew exactly how to care for Jerry. A mother of six, she fit into our lifestyle well. She was a committed Christian, too. Together the three of us managed nicely with help from Jennifer, Julie and the boys.

Dr. Loren stopped by one morning and had coffee with me. I was still in my gown. "You are O.K., aren't you? I don't understand it, but I can see that you are."

She went down to the re-creation room to see Jerry. They laughed and joked. She hadn't even brought in her little black bag; there was nothing medically she could do. She praised our hospital room setup and the way Jerry was being cared for. When she left, we hugged. "I love Jerry," she said softly.

"I know. He loves you too. He prays for you often and thanks God for you."

A couple of weeks later I called her with an emergency. Jerry's left leg had turned purple and there was obviously a blood clot: it was twice its normal size. Rose had it propped up on pillows. Jerry was confused and thought it was broken.

Dr. Loren gasped when she saw it. Then she motioned for me to step into another room. "I had no idea it was this bad. I'm afraid we may have to amputate."

No fear rose up in me. "No, we won't. He's not going to have to leave his home. God promised me that."

"I want him in the hospital," she said.

"No. It'll be all right. I promise. I know you're the doctor, but I know what I'm talking about."

"O.K, I'll give it two days and I'll stay in close touch with you. I want Rose and Jean to give Heparin injections in the stomach every twelve hours. I have to see almost immediate relief."

"You will," I promised.

She went in to tell him goodbye and asked the rest of us to leave the room. "I want to pray with him," she explained. We must have looked stunned. "I'm not a heathen like you all think," she said, "just because I can't talk openly about God like you do. I believe, too."

Within two days Jerry's leg was almost normal. Any movement at all was becoming harder, though, and we had to turn him often. He had one small pressure sore on the tip of his spine and we worked with it furiously until it almost disappeared. He never complained. Often I could see his mouth moving, singing along with the praise music. And when he couldn't do that, he'd raise one hand in praise. When I'd put it down, thinking he was asleep, he'd raise it again. It was becoming very difficult for him to speak. The corners of his eyelids were slightly torn from the pressure on his brain. He hiccupped sometimes all day long. His head was swelling at the spot where the tumor was. We shaved him, bathed him, put aftershave on him, joked with him, prayed with him, put him on the bedpan, held his hand, sang to him, and loved him. As long as he could talk he said, "Thank you, ladies. You are doing a mighty fine job."

We kept an accurate record of everything done for him those last six weeks. Medicines, baths, food, conversations, jokes, prayers, visitors. One remarkable entry was recorded on June 24, 1983. The event had actually occurred about a week before that, but Jerry had waited a while to share it. I remembered that night in mid-June when he was so very low that we all thought surely he was leaving us. Sometimes he had breathed only four times a minute. It was as though a giant factory was closing down under

orders and a few loyal employees simply would not quit. He'd
take one more breath. Then another. . . .

Once I had leaned over him, certain he was gone. But he
opened his eyes a little, and whispered, "Hiedy." It was during
this long, difficult night that Jerry had what is commonly termed
"a near death experience." What struck me so forcibly, when he
related it days later, was that Jerry had almost no imagination. He
could follow instructions to the letter, but he wasn't creative, nor
would he ever, ever exaggerate. He constantly got after me about
that: he was a stickler for facts. Jerry told the story first to Rose,
when he learned that she herself had had a near death experience.
She entered it in the record book; then he reported the experience
again for me, speaking softly because it was such an effort now
to talk. "I was on a train. A crowded train with lots of well
dressed people. All the people in my car were men—business-
men with briefcases. We realized that we were on our way to
heaven and we all felt excited. No fear. Then the train stopped,
and off in the distance we could see hell. We could feel the
intense heat, even though it was so far, and we could hear the
screams of the people. Everyone on the train wanted to move on.
It was so horrible." Jerry paused to rest.

Then he continued. "And then everyone on the train had to get
off. Everyone except three of us. I was one of the three who got
to stay on. The people who had to get off begged and screamed
and told about all the good works they had done on earth. I can
still seem to hear them screaming. And then the train moved on
. . . to heaven. I stood on a cloud and Jesus was on another
cloud. He looked at me with this wonderful look. Then He lifted
one finger like a football coach when he signals a boy to go into
the game. He reached across the clouds and drew me to Him
somehow. He told me, 'You almost missed this.' Then He said,
'I don't want you to stay right now. I want you to go back and tell
this experience.' He said that I should tell people that hell is very
real and even people in the church are going there. And He said
to tell people that heaven is very real too, but that you must know

Him personally to come in. He said that it's so simple, but that people keep refusing Him. He said that I had to tell this.''

Jerry looked directly at me and said, ''Mannie, you have to write it in the book. Will you? Do you believe me?''

''I will, and of course I believe you, Jer.''

He was very tired and went immediately to sleep. I sat beside him. It felt so good not to be afraid. Jerry knew I wasn't afraid and I knew he wasn't. It was our silent gift to each other. No fear. In a way Jerry had showed me how to live. And in a way I was helping him . . . to move on. I couldn't seem to think the word *death*. Every time I had to sign some kind of medical form that said ''terminal,'' I wanted to scratch through it and write ''transfer.'' And who am I to say that one doesn't get transferred by train? Anything's possible.

14

Tennis Shorts

On July 4th both Rose and Jean had family plans and Jerry and I were alone most of the day. I insisted that Jennifer go with Charlie on his family outing, and the boys were at our church's St. Simon's Island summer camp. Several people had said, "Surely you aren't going to let them go to camp. With their daddy . . . so near death. What if they aren't here?"

But I wasn't living with what-ifs anymore. The twins had wanted to go and I'd had peace about it. After I'd made the decision to allow them to go, the church phoned and said that a member who had a private plane would be on stand-by to bring them home, should they be needed. I was grateful. Jerry and I wanted our life to go on just as normally as possible.

He was sleeping most of the time now. There was not much to do for him unless he needed something for a headache. Before Jennifer and Charlie set out, I got them to help me put red, white and blue sheets on Jerry's bed to celebrate the Fourth. "Thanks," Jerry had managed. I sat by his bed holding his hand. He rallied about midday with an unusual request.

"I want my tennis shorts on." Maybe he was recalling that we were usually on vacation on the Fourth. I don't know what he was thinking. I had been remembering all the Fourths we'd spent in Florida: the fireworks, the beach, eating out, being sunburned.

I could see Jerry diving into the pool, swimming underwater and holding his breath "forever" until I'd be terrified. I remembered walking on the beach and holding hands. He usually bought new shorts for these vacations. I remembered what good legs he had, muscular and strong.

He made the request again. "Mannie, I want my tennis shorts on."

"Sure thing, Jer. It's a good idea." I pulled and tugged until I got his pajama bottoms off and the shorts on. It was a lot of work doing it alone. He'd lost so much weight that I had to tuck the shorts under him so they looked right.

"Thanks."

"You're welcome."

"You're going to hang in here all the way with me, aren't you, babe?"

"Yep, all the way. You can't get rid of me. I'm not about to miss the best part."

"I love you, Mannie. Lordy, how I love you. You're twenty-four carat gold."

"You're not exactly brass, yourself."

He was tired. I sat on the high stool by his bed, remembering. He patted my hand . . . to comfort me. That cut through unexpectedly. Tears came, and they felt good. It was only the third time I'd cried during this whole ordeal. I turned the fan up so he couldn't hear and continued sitting there holding his hand and crying.

Jerry was in such communion with Jesus that they seemed almost one. I felt left out, a little, but happy for him. Soon he'd be strong again, strong legs, leaping and running, praising God . . . in His very presence. The praise music that we kept going was playing softly. "Thou wilt keep him in perfect peace, whose mind is stayed on thee. . . ."

July 8th was my birthday. I had heard Jerry telling the girls to get me slacks and a blouse. I don't know how he was keeping up with the dates. The day after my birthday our Sunday school class had a picnic. It was only ten minutes from our house. Jerry wanted me to go and Rose did too and it felt right. The class had a big card for me and a birthday present and there were lots of smiles and hugs. Jennifer and my mother went with me and I thought, "I'm actually enjoying myself!"

It was thanks to the total relinquishment I had made of Jerry on May 11th. In order to do it I had to die to every dream, every right, every ambition. My life had to begin again. My neat little mapped-out future of growing old with Jerry had to be erased like a blackboard at the end of a school day. It was a tremendous price to pay for peace and joy, but it was the only way to be fear-free. Now I felt as though I were drifting down a lazy river with my hand hanging over the side of a boat. I'd go wherever the gentle river took me. No more struggling to go upstream against the current.

I was sleeping well, eating well, laughing some. The children were all O.K. My mother was with us. Jerry's folks came from time to time, but it was very difficult for them. Our cat often curled up at the foot of Jerry's bed. I remembered how Jerry hated cats when we married, but learned to tolerate and even love them because of my obsession with them. He was disgusted the first time I brought one home and said I couldn't name it something cute like "Bootsie" or "Butterball." "You name him, then," I beamed, excited that I could keep the kitten.

He thought for a while and finally announced, "Wingate. That's a no-nonsense name for a cat." Wingate lived with us for fifteen years.

Jerry didn't talk much now. But he still smiled and raised his hand in praise, and sometimes he spoke to us. I wanted him healed—transferred. I was almost impatient. All our married life I'd had to wait for him. Here I was waiting again. . . .

Once on a very difficult day when we couldn't seem to get Jerry comfortable—when he kept throwing up, when the headaches were impossible to get under control—I almost lost my joy for a moment.

"Lord, it's hard and ugly and loud and painful. Why is death so difficult?"

Birth is too, Marion. Remember the difficult delivery with your first child? It took thirty-six hours. Remember the pain? But it came to an end and you barely remember it now. You won't remember this after a while.

"I see, Lord. It's often hard to get into this world, and it's often difficult to get out. . . ."

15

Victory Sunday

It was Saturday, July 16th, a hot, muggy day. Jerry was so very weak and motionless that many times it seemed it was all over. I'd given him up so completely, that last breath didn't seem like a big deal somehow. He was in for such an adventure. I couldn't seem to think about my future without him. I just thought: he's almost well. God's Holy Spirit was everywhere in the re-creation room. There was no fear or defeat anywhere. Not a hint of it. We were smiling, even joking a little. The praise music was always going.

Around eleven o'clock that morning I asked some company to leave. It was the only time I'd done such a thing, but I wanted to be alone with Jerry one more time. I sat on the hospital bed and looked directly into his half-opened eyes. I couldn't help him breathe easier; still I had joy. I didn't understand it, but I held onto it. I began to sing along to the music; such joy welled up in me that I thought I might just float away. I talked to God out loud. He was so close. "Thank You, Father, oh, thank You. How I praise Your name. Thank You for the victory, the absence of fear. What You've taught both of us. What You are going to do with this situation—how You will somehow use it to Your glory. It is not for naught. Thank You for showing me how to relinquish Jerry to You. Thank You that we both know You and love You and trust You totally. Thank You that someday You'll show me how to write about this moment. . . ."

I was certain that Jerry understood. He tried to smile. I knew that he knew I was speaking for both of us. We were in perfect agreement.

I thought about Jerry's words just the day before. "I won." Winning had always been important to Jerry. He was competitive.

I thought about Julie bringing Jamie to visit Jerry just yesterday. Jamie was the same age I was when my father died. Jerry managed to say to her, "There's little Jamie. Sweet as ever." She was wearing a little ballerina dress and was dancing around his bed.

"See me, Grady, dancing for you!"

That Saturday morning I had asked Jon as he got ready to go to work at the meat market, "Jon, do you want to stay home today? Daddy will probably be going sometime today."

"No, ma'am. I want to go to work like always, and if it happens . . . I wish you wouldn't come get me. Just let me come home at my regular time."

"O.K., Jon." I trusted God to work out perfect timing so we'd all be here. Jon was better off working.

During the afternoon Rose and I stood together looking at Jerry as he slept and listened to the labored breathing. We were always grateful now for sleep. Suddenly we turned together and looked out the window into our front yard, where a sudden wind had sprung up. It had been such a still day that it startled both of us. Rose said, "Marion, the wind isn't blowing in anyone else's yard except yours!"

It was true. Only our trees tossed and swayed—the big maples Jerry had planted years ago. The wind came in the open window and blew our hair from our faces. It lasted less than two minutes. I was grateful that Rose had experienced the rushing of this sudden wind with me. We were even more certain of God's powerful presence and that Jerry's homegoing was imminent.

At ten-thirty that evening Rose and I lay down on the sofa bed

by Jerry's hospital bed. Jennifer stood at his bedside along with
our friend Jo Ann Thomason who had come that afternoon and
refused to leave. The boys and Mother had gone upstairs to bed.
Countless times we were certain that the end had come. Suddenly
I knew that Jerry'd be going to be with Jesus on a Sunday, early,
early, in the morning. How strange that I was dozing when Jerry
was taking his last breaths. How was that possible? The thing I'd
so feared was happening and I slept and peace was cemented in
my heart.

"Mama, Mama, come quick!"Jennifer called. "Daddy's going to Jesus now." I got up and came to Jerry's side. No panic.
No fear. I didn't even hurry. Mostly he had already gone. My joy
seemed to increase. The lights were not on in the re-creation
room, only in the hall. Jerry hadn't been able to move his head
to the left in weeks. Each time I had tried to help him turn it, he
cried out in pain. He had so wanted to turn it to the left. I reached
out and turned his head: it moved quickly and easily.

Rose hugged me. "Praise God, Marion. It's over." His skin
seemed to be getting white. Even in the dimly lit room. I didn't
look very much at his earth suit. In my mind I was seeing other
things—things of the spirit.

I remembered once watching an unwed mother give up her
baby for adoption. It was a tremendous act of love and I had
gotten caught up in her anguish. And then through a strange
series of events, I was involved in a small way in the lives of the
new adoptive parents and I experienced their joy—so intense I
thought my heart would burst.

God had spoken to me all those years ago: *This is like death for
a believer. It looks so horrible from one side, but remember the
rejoicing you have seen. Concentrate on the rejoicing. It's real.*

I remembered that powerful truth now and was hardly aware of
the quiet form on the hospital bed. I had forgotten how still death
could be. The absence of motion or sound was almost unbelievable. But I knew that now he was really moving as never before.
He was walking, running, laughing, rejoicing, singing, praising
our Father. His joy was complete, like his healing.

I can't remember ever being so excited except when our children were born. Jennifer was radiant. She ran to call Julie and in just a few moments Julie arrived, smiling and radiant too. Then someone called the undertaker, our friend Bob Frahm. When Bob walked in, he said, "I was up reading my Bible when the call came. The Lord had already told me that Jerry was coming to Him tonight."

He had left us at 12:45 A.M. Sunday morning, July 17. The other undertaker who came with Bob didn't know us and must surely have wondered at the smiles. "Is there anything special you want done, Mrs. West?" he asked with deep concern.

"Yes, we all want to ride in the hearse with you."

"I beg your pardon?"

"We rode in the ambulance after seizures so many times," I explained, "when there was no victory. We have the victory now and we want to make this victorious, fear-free ride."

Jerry had to be pronounced dead by a doctor before they could take him to a funeral home; it was a state law. Rose, Julie, Jennifer and I piled into the back of the hearse for the trip to the hospital. Dr. Loren was not on call and a very young doctor opened the back of the vehicle. "Oh my!" he said, jumping back as we all piled out. Then he looked cautiously inside and went on to do his pronouncing.

Back at home it was so late that Rose decided to bed down in my room for the rest of the night. Over and over we marvelled that Jerry was really and forever all right. The long ten-month battle was over. We had won! We switched off the light at about three-thirty in the morning.

An instant later I sat up. Rose did too. "What's that music?" I asked. "I don't know," Rose answered.

"The girls must be playing a tape," I said. Julie was staying over in Jennifer's room.

Just then Julie appeared in the doorway. "Mother, where's the music coming from?"

"We don't know," I answered. I'd switched off the praise tapes down in the re-creation room myself. Julie went back to bed, but I lay for a long time awake. The reality of Jesus and His victory was so magnificent that if a ten-foot angel had appeared, I think I simply would have said, "Hi there."

And still I could hear the mysterious music, even with the attic fan going. "Lord, what is it?" Now it was louder, clearer. I supposed everyone else in the house was asleep. I don't know Hebrew, but I heard a woman singing, chanting sort of, and I felt somehow it was Hebrew. After a few minutes many voices joined in singing with her. Right then I got another little mental picture. I could see a group of people in a circle. In the middle was Jerry, so happy and healthy, smiling that wonderful smile that seemed to give off light. From the beautiful music I can still remember one lovely word! It sounded like "Sone-yah." Very simply God seemed to say to me, *It's a welcome song, Marion. He's home now.*

Completely satisfied, I turned over and went to sleep.

16

The Promise

The funeral wasn't hard to face at all—so much easier than those days when the voices woke me up. People came by with food and flowers. I had asked Jerry Hutchins, the young man we'd met in the hospital, to sing "Blessed Assurance" and "It Is Well With My Soul." Jerry had to come from a town where he was preaching, a three-and-a-half hour drive, to sing for us.

While he was singing the second song I thought about Horatio Spafford, the man who wrote that hymn back in the 1800s. He composed it after learning that his four daughters had drowned in a shipwreck. I listened to the words: "When peace like a river attendeth my way, when sorrows like sea billows roll, whatever my lot, thou hast taught me to say, it is well, it is well with my soul. . . ."

Why, Horatio Spafford had entered into Nevertheless Living a hundred years ago. He may have called it something else, but he'd surely made the same astonishing discovery that I had. And Paul must have too, as he sat in prison singing. And Noah . . . building such a big boat far from the water. Thousands and thousands must have made this discovery before me.

In the room at the funeral home where the closed coffin was,

I'd kept the praise music going. I'd brought the tape from home: "By His word there is no fear in me . . . I've been set free. . . ."

When our family first went to "view the body," some were concerned that I might fall apart. Instead, when I looked down for a brief instant I had the feeling that I might smile or even laugh. It wasn't Jerry. He was long gone! That's when I had the coffin shut. All the family members were in agreement.

I didn't want any flowers on the coffin Jon had selected. It was magnificent, very simple. We ordered a dozen red roses and they stood on a table with a picture of Jerry when he coached a basketball team, and Jerry's marked-up Bible.

More than four hundred people attended the service. Many came up afterward and said their lives had been changed. During his remission, when Jerry thought he was getting well, he'd talked about going into the ministry. He was well and he was ministering.

At the cemetery in Elberton, our parents' home, I hugged old friends who hadn't been able to get to Atlanta for the funeral. It was almost one hundred degrees and many of those attending the burial were elderly. Some had taught Jerry and me in high school, some in Sunday school. I had ordered his marker. Of course it wasn't there yet, but it would say:

JERRY MICHAEL WEST
April 9, 1935–July 17, 1983
"More than a conqueror
through Christ Jesus
Who loved us" (Romans 8:37)

Oddly enough, in the days that followed I didn't experience a great sense of loneliness. I could concentrate, write thank you notes. Six o'clock had lost its terror. Living without Jerry somehow wasn't anything compared to the *fear* of living without him. I was a new person. I hardly knew me. The old Marion had died on May 11th. She had to die, so I could go on living. I didn't want her to reappear. She had been so fearful and full of self-pity and despair.

Mail poured in, much of it from *Guideposts* readers who had learned of Jerry's death. Many of the letters said something like, "I've never been religious or even read the Bible, but my mother sends me *Guideposts*. When I read your story about Jerry, I just bowed my head and asked Jesus into my life. . . . I can't tell you all that's happened to me. It's so different with Him in charge."

The mailwoman rang my doorbell one day and asked, "Who are you? Why do you get so much mail?"

When I explained she said, "But you don't look sad or anything. My father just died and my mother is going to pieces."

I explained the basics of Nevertheless Living and she asked, "Could my mother call you? Would you tell her too?"

I gave away all of Jerry's things. The children, of course, took what they wanted. Jennifer's boyfriend, Charlie, chose some suits. Then a missionary from India came to speak at our home Bible study, which I was continuing. He was a medical doctor working with lepers, prostitutes and orphans. When I offered him some of Jerry's clothes tears sprang up in his eyes. "They are so needed. Could I have everything in the closet?"

Someone from Georgia Power brought all the things from Jerry's office. There was a big box of awards and recognitions that he'd gotten through the years and never even mentioned or hung up or brought home. There were pictures of him that I'd never seen, taken at work, smiling as usual.

I didn't have the sensation some people do when a loved one dies, that the person could walk in at any time. I was grateful for that. I did have to learn to control my thoughts in order not to relive the bad parts . . . the details of sickness. My mind wanted to go over and over them, but I battled not to think about things that would do me no good.

I could see that I was going to have time and energy to write and speak again. Since I was no longer afraid I had more energy for everything! People even said I looked different. Several years before, when I'd been pounding away at the typewriter most of the day, accepting speaking invitations right and left, I could feel the resentment building up in Jerry, and in the children, too. Jerry would encourage me to write and speak, but it often caused a wall between us. He denied it but I was pretty good at spotting walls. So one day I told God that I had to give it all up. "I can't handle both, Lord. You see I can't. Right now I want to concentrate on being a wife and mother." I had added almost as an afterthought, "If I ever have another life to live, I'll write and speak again. But I can't now. Thank You for letting me do it for ten years. It was a dream come true. A gift from You."

I never told my family about that decision, I was just home more. Things were better organized. The typewriter got dusty and the cat began to sleep on it.

Now suddenly here I was in my forties, without a husband, one daughter married, another about to be married, and two teenage sons. Looked like I could write again.

Jerry had made me promise to do a book about what we'd learned through his illness. I had no idea how to write such a book, but that was nothing new. I thought of my first book, *Out of My Bondage*, published in 1976. I had written it with Jon and Jeremy crawling all over me; two little girls who needed lots of attention and a husband who thought I was wasting my time. Only Julie had encouraged me. She was nine years old and came in from school each day, put her books down and asked, "Where's the book, Mom? Let me read some more." That's all the encouragement I had, but it was enough. Somehow I finished the book and actually landed a contract, which I never read. I just signed it.

The holdup was that Jerry would not allow me to send in the final few chapters or return the contract until he checked over what I'd written about him. "Please read it, Jerry," I'd beg nightly.

"O.K.," he'd say.

But he didn't read it and for three weeks, which seemed like three years, it lay untouched. I had no way of understanding that Jerry was afraid of what people might think about him . . . and me. That I might be ridiculed. No one else's wife was writing a book with a title like *Out of My Bondage*. They were driving car pools, exchanging recipes and doing needlepoint. I had almost hated him as he sat there reading the sports page. One evening I went upstairs, locked myself in the bathroom, fell down on the floor and cried out to God, "O Father, I love that book. I don't even know how I got it written. *I have a contract!* Me, a nobody who can't even spell. And now he's not going to let me return it. Help me somehow to give up the book and not be mad at him. I don't understand why he doesn't want me to write."

After the tears stopped, I washed my face and went downstairs to fix supper. Jerry came into the kitchen with a look of anguish and love on his face: "You can mail the contract and I approve of the chapters. I can't hold you back. It's good. God said for me to stop holding you back. Your book is good, Marion."

I ran into his arms and must have clung to him for a full five minutes. He added, "I hope this is the only one." It hadn't been the only one—and now it was Jerry himself who'd committed me to yet another.

But . . . how big a truth did I really have to share? The Nevertheless Principle had brought me through the crisis of Jerry's illness and death. Would it stand up in the dry dailyness of living alone? That was what I had to set out to discover.

17

Fear

One thing I learned at the outset: Nevertheless Living is never automatic. Fear would try again and again to reenter my life. It had been there for so long that it must have missed its comfortable haven. I still thought of it as that angry little gray man who had to go.

Jerry had been gone less than a week when it tried literally to sneak back through a window. The summer screens! Though he'd talked about it for years, Jerry had never had the old, worn window screens replaced. Now fear suggested, "Your house will probably fall apart. You don't know how to take proper care of things. Look at those screens." I knew I had to win that battle right then.

"Boys," I called out, "take down one of the big screens and one of the small ones and we'll take them to the store." It was the Saturday after Jerry died; he and the boys always tackled some kind of home improvement project on Saturdays.

"Just measure them, Mom, No one takes the screens to the store."

"No. I never measure right, and I don't trust your measuring either."

"Aw, Mom," both boys wailed.

"I'm waiting in the car." They appeared, each carrying a

different sized screen. We drove to the best hardware store in the area. All the way I prayed, "Lord, let some nice old man help us, who has all day and won't ask hard questions. Don't let anyone snap at me."

Jon and Jeremy dropped the screens on the counter and moved away from the situation. An elderly man, the very image of Captain Kangaroo, came up. "Good morning. May I help you, ma'am?"

"Yes, I need some screens. I don't know how to measure so I brought my old ones." He picked up the screens with a nod of approval. "Won't make a mistake when you bring them in, will you?"

"I need three of the small ones and seven of the big ones." Our transaction was over in less than five minutes. I felt marvelous. No reason to be afraid of replacing screens.

Far worse was my fear of balancing the checkbook. For twenty-five years I'd messed it up. Jerry always lectured to me before bailing me out. It was the same lecture year after year: "Marion, when you write a check to Big Apple Food Store, you can't just draw an apple and expect me to understand. And when you write checks, you subtract, you don't add!"

In the final months of his illness I'd been letting the statements pile up, not even opening them. One morning after he died I knew I was about to be afraid of them. So I took all the statements and went to our bank. The friendly woman at the desk smiled, "May I help you?" I laid seven statements on her desk.

"I can't do bank statements." She knew about Jerry. "We'll have your account straight in no time," she said encouragingly. Just make a copy of your checkbook entries. Come back tomorrow and we'll have your correct balance."

Weeks later, three women were still working on my statements. The bank officer told me, "Mrs. West, we may have to close down your account and open a new one."

"That's O.K. We've had to do that before. I expected that."

I didn't understand about investing money, either. Anything over five hundred dollars confused me. Julie and our lawyer,

Lendon Gibbs, were getting discouraged trying to explain dividends and interest to me. The more they added up figures and talked to me in that patient, surely-you-can-understand-this voice, the more I wanted to run from the room. "Mother," said Julie. "It's like if you have a lot of jelly beans and you keep putting them in a big jar. When you want a few jelly beans you go to the jar and take some out."

I looked over at Lendon. He had been our friend for more than twenty years. He and Jerry worked together and thought alike.

"Do whatever you think best with the money. Do what Jerry would do. I don't have to understand this right now. I trust you."

Lendon nodded and Julie looked relieved. I felt a surge of contentment. I didn't have to learn everything at once. God would put people in my life to help me. Driving home, Julie said, "How do you feel?"

"I want some jelly beans," I said. We stopped and I bought a big bag of jelly beans and we ate them all.

I could have easily panicked about the income tax. Even with Jerry doing it, it was always an ordeal for me. My job was to keep receipts, checks, etc., for the entire year. He filled out all the forms and all I had to do after I got the stuff together was to sign "Marion Bond West" on a line that he showed me. Even this past spring when he'd been so ill, he'd managed to do it. His handwriting was different, and it took him five times as long, but he did it.

I was learning to turn to God at the first prickle of fear, so I prayed, "Father, I need a woman who knows how to do taxes to come spend the day at my house. She needs to have a sense of humor and be a Christian and be very patient and not fuss at me."

Someone to whom I confided my prayer recommended a young mother with two small children. She appeared at my front door two weeks later at eight-thirty in the morning. "Hi, Marion," she smiled. "I'm going to do your taxes."

I watched her in amazement. She made phone calls like Jerry, wrote down numbers and percentages. She searched under the bed with me and helped me ransack drawers and must have said fifty times, "It's going to be all right. Relax."

She even agreed to take the forms home to finish when it was time to pick her husband up at work. I went to bed thinking: The taxes are done! They're really done. How did she know what to do? I keep Cindy's number over my phone where most people keep police and fire department numbers.

The secret, I was learning, was to throw Nevertheless victory at the fear before it ever got started. Doing this, I even overcame my lifelong horror of getting lost. Before, when I had three errands to do in a day, I often came all the way back home and started over because I only knew how to get somewhere from my house, not how to cut across the expressway. I marvelled over my friends who could drive their husbands to the airport. Jerry would never have dreamed of asking me to do that. Now, I ventured to new places and sure enough made all the wrong turns—but I wasn't afraid. "I'm lost again, Father. Nevertheless, You know where I am." I'd stop and ask directions, laughing at my own stupidity. "One day, Lord, I'm actually going to drive to the Atlanta airport."

I had about decided to sell the freezer because it was full of ice and I'd never defrosted it. It had been Jerry's purchase: I had never wanted one. But I knew I mustn't let myself be afraid of defrosting a freezer, and anyway I couldn't sell it full of ice. So I walked up to it, opened the door and said, "Nevertheless, I'm not afraid of you." Of course people got tired of hearing about my defrosting prowess. I even made long distance calls to tell about the achievement.

I had the house painted, selected new wallpaper, bought a new refrigerator and learned that you must have the oil checked in the car. Buying new tires was a must too, even if the old ones still rolled around.

Then I did something I thought I could never do: I taught Jon and Jeremy to drive. I was learning that the minute I wanted to back away from something, that was the minute I had to face it.

When the furnace went out in the middle of an extremely cold night, instead of panicking I called out to the boys to get it going. Jon tried first, but couldn't do it. Then Jeremy went down and called up the steps, "Mama, it won't light."

"You have to learn to do it," I called back from my warm bed. "Are you praying?"

"You can't pray about a furnace. It's mechanical."

"Nevertheless, I'm praying."

Maybe two more minutes passed, while Jeremy continued to grumble and bang the furnace. Then a big "whoosh" as it came on. Jeremy came bounding up the steps, "Mama, Mama, I prayed and it worked! It really works. You can pray about a furnace."

I began to speak to groups about fear and one day I happened to mention that at one time I'd been afraid to go to the mailbox . . . because the insurance forms might be there. I'd always been afraid of filling in blanks. I hated to open the box and find those forms. Afterward a woman came up in tears. "Honey, I've been afraid of the mailbox for so long . . . ever since my husband died. I was afraid to tell anyone because they might think I was crazy. I want to be fear-free, too."

That day many women confessed their deep fears. "I'm afraid of the dark." "I'm afraid of my husband." "I'm afraid of dying." And so I shared with them the fear I'd had to overcome to be there at all. The fear of speaking in public. . . .

18

The Outline

I remembered so clearly my first speaking encounter. It was in 1976 when I was invited to come back to my home church in Elberton, Georgia, where I'd grown up, and speak to a few ladies in the library—just ten or twelve old friends.

The fear was enormous. I had never spoken in front of a group. I could barely manage to read the minutes in a club where I held the office of recording secretary. But the invitation was so warm that I thought: these are old and dear friends; some are so elderly that they won't pay much attention to what I say anyway. I can have it all written out and read it like minutes from a meeting.

Still I prayed that it would snow and I'd have to cancel the engagement. But the temperature that February day was in the 70s. When I arrived at the church the ladies met me in the parking lot and said we were going to have the meeting in Fellowship Hall instead of the library. One of them explained, "We put a little article in the paper, Marion, and a few more people than we expected showed up." I peeked in and it looked like the entire town of Elberton sat there. I almost turned and ran. *If I could only faint,* I thought. I even had a wild hope that the Rapture would occur.

Someone was introducing me, telling what a bright little girl I had been. As the applause died away I stood before what looked like to me all the people in the world. My hands were shaking so I could hardly hold my speech and my vision was so blurred I couldn't see the paper anyway. Quickly, and silently I heard from God: "Forget about your written speech. That's what *you* want to say, anyway. Say what I tell you to say, even though you don't understand. Trust Me."

I made a decision. "You're on, God. Let's go." I stuck the speech in the back of my Bible and looked out at the people. Thoughts came to me as if on ticker tape. Often I didn't even know the end of a sentence till I got there. I talked for over an hour without a trace of nervousness. I never planned to speak again, but for seven years, I told those women on the day we shared our fears, I'd been standing up and thoughts had come to me as I said them, never knowing what the next thought would be.

I was making another discovery about Nevertheless Living, though. Not only is it not automatic—it's never static, either. Soon after I shared this story, God used another speaking date to heal a still deeper fear.

This time the call was from the minister of a church in a nearby town. "Would you conduct workshops for us after you speak?"

I'd never done a workshop in my life, but I felt God telling me to accept. *Just agree,* came the powerful thought. "I don't know how to do a workshop," I told him over the phone. "And I never plan ahead what I'll say. I'll do it if you're comfortable with that."

"Certainly. Just send us an outline. It's sort of a formality— just to let the ladies know what to expect. You don't actually have to stick right to it."

I hung up and thought, *O Lord, I can't do an outline!* I didn't even make outlines when I wrote books. Outlines are like bank statements. In the bed a sneaky fear of creating an outline began to torment me. *I can't be afraid of an outline, I've come too far for that.* I turned on the light. It was eleven P.M. and I'm usually asleep by ten, but I was wide awake. I got out paper and pen and began making notes. It was after midnight when I turned out the

light. The outline looked like a real outline with Roman numerals
and all. I didn't actually plan to use it, but at least I'd have
something to submit to them. I turned off the light no longer
afraid of an outline, and went immediately to sleep.

At three A.M. I woke up, the outline vivid in my mind. The
points concerned the healing of childhood memories and becoming free of fear. Maybe it wasn't so silly after all. Maybe it was
a real outline. And then a list began forming in my mind. I didn't
understand it at first: it was names of people, some of whom I
knew well, some I could barely remember, and others I'd never
met. All were men or boys. My grandfather's name headed the
list. I'd never known him; he died when my father was a boy.
Then my father's name appeared, then a brother who was still-
born. There were twenty-six names in all. "What does it mean,
Lord?"

Gently God explained that in some way or another I had felt
rejection in my subconscious from all these people. To a little girl
not yet two, the death of a father came across as abandonment.
So did the lack of a grandfather and a brother. Why, I had deep
roots of rejection and never knew it! Now God wanted to heal this
list so that there would be no possibility that I could ever add
Jerry to it. I was certain, too, that God wanted me to talk about
the list at the workshop.

I got out of bed and wrote down all the names on the list.
Staring at it, I understood why I had trouble relating to certain
men. Why sometimes, when I phoned a friend and her husband
answered, I'd have to fight the urge to hang up.

A long-forgotten memory surfaced. I was playing paper dolls
on the floor of my mother's closet. I loved paper dolls, you could
pretend anything, have a father. I leaned to the left and was
surprised to learn that the closet went back farther than I suspected. I pushed the dresses aside and moved back into the secret
area and found a pair of my father's boots and some trousers. An
intense feeling welled up inside me. I held the shoes and the
pants. I even tried the boots on. It was something of my father to
hold onto. Looking at those boots, another memory had come. I

was in the bathroom in my diapers, not much taller than the toilet. I was playing in the toilet and reached up and pulled the handle. A big sound came and I saw some water. A pair of boots, the same boots I had found in the closet, appeared. I could not remember above my father's knees. He had on khaki pants tucked into the tan boots and I held onto his pants.

I loved to crawl back in the closet and play with the boots. I could remember when he actually wore them! Back in that closet was like another world to me, like the Father's Day card. I pretended that I sat on his lap, like the little girl on the card.

I believed all of this—the list, the memory—was opening up because Jerry had helped me to say "Daddy." Now I understood a little more about why I'd been so unreasonable with Jerry, why I constantly wanted him to talk to me and tell me that he loved me. It was this pattern of imagined rejection—unrecognized, undealt with.

The next day I phoned the pastor and read part of my outline to him. The speech and workshop weren't for a number of months, so I put it out of my mind and promptly misplaced the outline. Meanwhile I began attending seminars on the healing of painful memories and reading books, and although I didn't see myself as a counselor, God seemed to give me answers when I talked with people. Many women, it seemed, were angry with their fathers for having left them through death or divorce—angry and afraid. I noticed that when someone confided something to me that had happened at age five, she would, in many ways, resemble a five-year-old child. Her gestures, even her speech patterns would change, showing how alive that little girl was in the grown woman.

When the minister from out of town called to confirm my speaking engagement, I confessed to him that I'd lost my outline.

"Oh, my word! Don't tell my wife. She'll have a nervous breakdown. She's an outline person. Very organized. She's worked so hard on this seminar."

Sure enough, a few days before the workshop someone handed me their denominational newspaper, which went all over the South. There was an announcement of the workshop and my partial outline. I felt like running and saying to God, "See what they've done? They've printed part of that outline that I lost and didn't even understand. What will I do?"

Instead I heard myself say aloud, "Nevertheless, Father, I am going to trust You." I wasn't afraid . . . of failure . . . of making a fool of myself . . . of looking ridiculous. "I love not being afraid, Lord. I want to help others not be afraid too."

When I reached the church, however, my confidence faltered. "Lord, are You certain You want me *here*? I mean, they all look so together. They're smart dressers, perfect makeup. See them laughing and talking—they don't look afraid of anything."

They filled the entire church auditorium. All smiling with their hands in their laps. Notebooks and pens in their laps, too. Someone introduced me and I stood there and said something like, "I don't have an outline or notes and I have no idea what will happen today. None of you looks like you have any problems . . . but you must because God only sends me where women are hurting. Some of you are hurting so badly you dare not let the frozen smiles off your faces. God wants me to talk to you about Nevertheless Living. He wants to bring about healing in your lives today. What He has for you will be available only to those of you who are desperate. He only works with people who can't handle things on their own any longer. God never has helped those who help themselves. Benjamin Franklin was wrong about that."

I shared some of my testimony, beginning with when Jerry and I were dating. I spoke for an hour and a half. Then since 300 women were there I taught three consecutive workshops. If I'd had an outline I would have done the same workshop three times, but since I had no notes I taught three different ones, going a bit deeper each time. My favorite part was the question-answer time. I didn't have the answers to most of the questions, but my Father did and He gave them to me quickly and faithfully.

That same day I drove to another town and spoke for five hours and prayed and talked with women for two hours more and had no sensation of being tired. It simply was not I. I was even relaxed enough to teach with my shoes off. The beautiful women wearing the right colors were like women everywhere . . . hurting, afraid, even terrified. Many had lived through experiences no one would ever imagine. The hurts came pouring out and I never for a moment considered that people were asking me for help, but rather the Helper.

It was one of the most memorable experiences of my life. I marvelled how God can use anyone. I believe in people being trained, I believe in college and seminaries and degrees and preparing yourself. But I also believe a quote from Elbert Hubbard I read once in *Guideposts*: "God will not look you over for medals, degrees or diplomas, but for scars."

I guess I qualified and now He was showing me how scars could be used. I hated for the day to end. Driving home I kept thinking: "I wasn't afraid, Lord. No fear." I crawled into bed, but I was too buoyed up to sleep.

I got back up and decided to look through the day's mail. There were several letters from people I didn't know. I read one with special excitement. There have been many such letters now, but this was the very first.

"Marion, I was full of fear of being alone because I knew my husband was planning to leave me and our children, and he did. I planned at different times to take my life. He left us over a woman. I never knew pain could go so deeply. I had a lot of Bible knowledge in my head, but there was almost nothing in my heart. Thank you for your last letter. I never realized the word *nevertheless* was in the Bible, let alone so many times, until you pointed it out. Nevertheless Living works! My favorite is Psalm 106:8. 'Nevertheless, you saved them—to defend the honor of your name and demonstrate your power to all the world.' I believe now that God is going to save this situation. I have gone from crying over his leaving us, to relief that he was finally gone, to hating him for doing this to us, to wanting him back so badly that I could hardly stand it.

"Today, however, I stand firm on the belief that God will deliver us into a godly marriage. My heart is lonely for my husband, but my faith in God is strong. Sometimes it is so strong that I actually wonder if I'm a little on the wacky side because I truly believe! Our marriage is hopeless in the eyes of the world, but with spiritual eyes I see plenty of hope. This is a very scattered letter written on my knees as I sit in a swing and listen to my seven-year-old's continuous talking. Thank you for telling me about Nevertheless Living.''

And thank you, I thought, *for showing me that it works for others.* This deserted wife was on her way all right: feeling a little wacky—even being accused of being wacky—is often one of the first signs of entering into Nevertheless Living!

How does it work? What had I actually done at the workshop not to feel any pressure? I remembered something Julie said once. I used to dread going into a mall because so many things distracted me and I could never concentrate on what I'd come to get. Julie had come up with an answer. ''Mama, just get in a bubble and float in and float out. You won't be aware of anything except what you're there for. Nothing can touch you in a bubble. I get in them all the time when I have to do hard things.'' By applying her childlike formula I learned to run in and out of a mall in ten minutes. It works in grocery stores, too.

Now I saw that the notion had a spiritual application. Once I heard a minister in Florida, Peter Lord, describe something similar. He said that when you have to do something difficult, you need to get *into* Jesus! He emphasized ''into.'' He said that most of us just go to Jesus, even lean on Him, but that in some situations this was not enough. ''Get inside Jesus . . . not just close to Him. Then He takes *all* the pressure. And believe me He knows how to take pressure. You don't have to feel a thing.'' He had drawn a square and a stick figure and then put the stick figure inside the square. ''See, get into Jesus.''

Inside the bubble of Jesus, I thought lying in bed, almost asleep, nothing can disturb your peace. I drifted off to sleep and the last thought I had was that Jesus gives you joy, nevertheless.

19

Thoughts

I woke up early the next morning. Thoughts were coming so fast that I ran to the typewriter. Very quietly like a sunrise God was telling me something about joy. It seemed to be in the form of a poem. I never write poetry. But I typed fast, having no idea what the next line would say.

THE CHOICE

We have to make a choice
To live in despair
Or joy
To walk in fear
Or in faith
To dwell under the shadow of the Almighty
Or reside in open spaces of self-effort
There's no in-between place
No half-way house
It's one way or the other
Pity for ourselves
Or compassion for others
Loneliness

Or reaching out
Joy and happiness are not even related
Joy springs from deep within
And has nothing to do with circumstances
Jesus promised us His joy
Happiness comes from without
Through things, people, desires fulfilled
Help me, Father, for I have made a choice
Not based on emotion
I have chosen to reject despair, fear and finally
Self-pity
Looking to you alone . . .
Oh, Father, already I sense the joy that comes
From the agonizing choice I made.

After I finished I sat and read and reread it. The poem did not come from me. I didn't know that I could deliberately determine what I thought about. That I could consciously refuse fear-thoughts and envy thoughts—and that when I did not, the enemy could gain precious ground. *Your thought life,* God seemed to be saying, *is this month's schoolroom in Nevertheless Living.*

Sure enough, every book I picked up, every Bible study I attended in the next few weeks, zeroed in on thoughts. In one place I read that we have only five seconds to refuse a thought. If we don't do it then, it has gained entrance to our minds. I began to see that I must identify where thoughts come from. I went to one seminar where the teaching "happened" to be on fantasies. I'd never thought about fantasy being important. But a memory came. . . . After Jerry and I were married, when he didn't give me the constant attention that I expected, I found a way of escape that I thought was harmless enough: daydreams about a boy I'd dated before Jerry and I were serious. I allowed "innocent" thoughts about this person from my past to drift casually through my mind. I was certain now they were well-aimed fiery darts from the enemy. Such little thoughts at first! Remembered fun. Nothing serious. Then one night I dreamed about this person. I'd never had a dream like that before. The next morning I told Jerry while he shaved. I was certain I'd get his attention then. "Um hum." He went off to work whistling. He wasn't even jealous!

Angry with him, I began to concentrate on the old boyfriend. It was a gradual thing, but it became a powerful part of my life. I thought: *What if I had married him?* I imagined what he'd be like as a husband. Of course he never watched television or read the sports page. He gave me loads of attention. It wasn't until I discovered I was pregnant with twins, and there was no room in my thoughts for anything else, that the fantasies about the former boyfriend stopped.

Listening at the seminar, I realized how perilous my position had been. A fantasy, the speaker explained, nearly always starts innocently enough, with a tiny, seemingly random thought. Satan is extremely patient. He will spoonfeed us wrong thoughts for months, even years, to bring about wrong action. I suspect that most of the time murder begins with the thought of revenge. A runaway wife or husband must mentally live through the "big escape" for a long time, going over and over the alluring aspects. Satan is careful not to show the anguish involved. He came to rob, steal and destroy. That's his evil goal. To cause dissension in churches, anger and bitterness between marriage partners, deception between children and parents, silence and apathy between neighbors and relatives. We don't battle flesh and blood but the tearing down of strongholds . . . mental strongholds that hold us in bondage, sometimes for a lifetime.

I knew that the first Christmas without Jerry was going to be a major testing ground for my new, disciplined thought life. For months beforehand the enemy kept reminding me of the previous one, the Christmas I thought I could not live through, trying to get me to dwell on the agony of it. Again and again I refused such broodings.

Remember how you were afraid of a Christmas tree? fear suggested. *What if you never have the courage to have another one?*

I shot back, "Nevertheless, we are going to have a tree. In fact we just might have two!"

The formerly vicious enemy of what-if crept off, limping. Early in December I purchased a small tree and put it on a little pine table that stands in the center of my kitchen. I decorated it with red calico bows and small artificial red apples. Enthused with the little kitchen tree, I crawled up into the attic and pulled out other decorations. I praised God because I wasn't afraid of Christmas; I put on Christmas music and sang as I worked.

Somehow I hit upon the idea of having a fancy dinner party just for my children. I'm sure the idea must have been from God. Last year the holidays had been so painful that I wanted this year's to be special for them. I set the table in the kitchen with great care in red and green, with handmade placecards. I got out the real silver and crystal and bought candles. I had candles all over the kitchen.

There had been some criticism of how I was spending money by one of my children. I thought I had been doing pretty well, but one child especially didn't think things were fair. Besides that, the boys had asked for really large gifts this year. I didn't like that and they knew it. Even when Jerry was alive it always seemed pagan to me to buy gifts for each other when we had so much. I wanted to help someone really needy, or use the money for missions. "You're being selfish," I had protested when the twins presented their "wish list." I thought about not getting them anything. I was praying aloud about the matter at Bible study one night when a friend interposed. "Marion, your boys are still hurting. They equate gifts with love right now. It will pass. Get them the things they want, even if they are excessive. This is a special Christmas, they need something extra. In fact, why not some extra spending money, so *they* can go all out on Christmas buying too?"

I knew the advice was from God. Before our dinner party I went to the bank: As I set the table I slipped a hundred dollar bill under each plate.

I cooked all the traditional foods. The house looked wonderful and the table was beautiful. The little tree looked very victorious. Looks of surprise crossed each child's face as he or she came into the kitchen.

"Gee, Mom."

"It's beautiful."

"Wow."

"You must have worked hard."

We all sat down and ate and everyone talked at once and there was laughter. When I told them to look under the plates there were more looks of astonishment . . . and gratitude.

The following week the children picked out the big tree for the living room. We decorated it together like people do on the Christmas television specials, and no one said one word of criticism.

The only thing I refused to do was hang up stockings and stuff them. I had never really enjoyed that, but the children loved it and Jerry always asked me to do it one more year. This year I gave advance notice: "No stockings."

"Aw, Mom," everyone said. Even Julie.

I wasn't going to do it, though. Then shortly before Christmas an enormous package arrived from a *Guideposts* reader whom I knew only through letters. She had asked the children's names and ages and I thought maybe she was going to send them personalized book markers. When I opened the huge box and pulled away mounds of tissue paper there I found beautiful red-checked Christmas stockings, perhaps two feet long. Each stocking had a name on it, and there was one for me too! Oh, I was so excited; no wonder the children liked stockings so much. And each stocking was crammed full of wrapped gifts. It was such a labor of love that my eyes brimmed with tears. I knew this woman was going through a crisis comparable to my own—and she didn't even know us. But my loving Father knew my children needed those stockings. And here they were. I hid them until Christmas Eve.

Often during those weeks I had to go back to the same drug store where the year before I'd stood in line getting prescriptions filled for Jerry. I looked at greeting cards casually, even the ones that said "Husbands," and my joy remained intact. I bought wrapping paper, ribbon, Scotch tape, cards and hummed along with the Christmas music that filled the store. Someone gave me some good advice once. When you lose something dear, concentrate on what you have left. I had lost something dear indeed; nevertheless I was rich.

There was another battle for my thought life as 1983 ended, one that had nothing to do with Christmas. I had not been back to the cemetery in Elberton since the day of the funeral five months earlier, which meant I had not seen Jerry's marker. Memories of myself as a little girl going to my daddy's grave in the same cemetery came to my mind. Before 1984 began, I knew I should go to see Jerry's marker. It wasn't that I had any sense of Jerry's being there; I simply didn't want to let fear of a grave marker find any growing-room in my thoughts. On my Christmas trip home to Elberton I went to the cemetery alone. I walked up the granite steps and looked down at the marker. I had designed it and it was just as I envisioned it. I only looked for a few moments. No great emotions swept over me. Now I had seen it. I certainly wasn't afraid of it. I walked away and haven't been back. I've offered to go with the children, but so far none of them has expressed a desire to go. Jerry simply isn't there. If they choose to never go, it's O.K. with me.

All of us were together on Christmas morning. Julie and Ricky came over with Jamie. Everyone was speechless over the stockings. Julie seemed to especially enjoy the dinner. With a new baby on the way, she always seemed to be hungry. Charlie was with us. Jennifer wore the diamond he had given her and they planned to be married in September.

I was ready for 1984. At one point during 1983 I had felt like the tiny kitten I'd found once. A dog had shaken it almost to death. As I held it gently, it played dead, refusing to move or respond. But gradually the weakened kitten learned to trust again. It lifted its head, looked around, stood on wobbly legs. The kitten had survived the attack, just as I had survived. Whatever 1984 held, I determined to remain on my Island of Trust, allowing fear-thoughts no access. Whatever could happen would never be as bad as being afraid of it.

I was progressing in the school of Nevertheless. But always there were further lessons, more to learn. If fear was a constant temptation to venture from my island, self-pity was another—and it was strongest when I was tired or feeling discouraged. That's a favorite time for the enemy to assault our thought lives, proposing the ideas he is programming for us. One afternoon in January, six months after Jerry's death, he attacked almost before I realized what was happening. I was alone and he sprang like a beast jumping on a dozing animal. Soon I knew I was in a battle, but I didn't feel like struggling. I wanted just to give in to self-pity. I deserved to feel sorry for myself now and then. Depression entered my bedroom like a living presence, bringing a whole train of suggestions from Satan:

Where are all my good friends now? I can't really write. No one is encouraging me. I'll never write another book. I miss being a wife. I miss being loved. I miss laughing. I . . . I . . . I . . . poor suffering me. Bless my hurting heart. No one really understands. My children are critical of me. I may just give up the Christian walk. Certainly I won't go to the Bible study tonight.

Maybe Nevertheless Living wasn't a reality, after all. Maybe it was just a word.

20

The Rescue

It was four-thirty that January afternoon when the attack came. Before long not only was I wallowing in self-pity, but I was wretchedly aware that my joy was gone.

When I was a little girl my cat, Josephine, had a litter of kittens. While the mother cat was outside one day, I moved the kittens to a warmer spot. When Josephine came back in the house the kittens were gone. She ran from one room to another meowing frantically. Finally, I caught her. She struggled in my arms, but I managed to hold onto her until I could place her in the box with her kittens. Instantly she purred with relief and nestled down in the cardboard box. She looked at me almost with apology in her yellow eyes as if to say: I should have trusted you.

Now I felt like Josephine. Where was my victory—my joy? It must be somewhere. How could I find it again? *Please don't let this happen, God.* I remembered the depression and hopeless feelings that had held me in a vise for so long. The phone rang and I grabbed for it. Maybe it was help.

Please be help, I prayed silently.

"Hi, Marion. It's Philip."* I hadn't seen Philip in a while, but

* (real names not used)

he was a minister and I just knew he was going to offer help. Only thing is, he sounded almost as desperate as I felt.

"Listen, there's a lady in my office right now named Belle Williams* who says she knows you. She . . . er . . . needs a place to stay tonight. It's almost dark and we don't have facilities to. . . ."

I remembered Belle: thin, desperate, apologetic, twisting her hands nervously, chain-smoking. She'd probably been pretty once. I'd known her for a number of years, and sometimes talked to her about Jesus. She was an abused wife who'd had to be hospitalized after severe beatings. She'd been in and out of drug and alcoholic rehabilitation centers. I suppose she had the lowest self-esteem of anyone I'd ever known. The horrors of her life piled up until one almost couldn't believe any one person had lived through so much hurt and humiliation. She had been dumped on the street now and had found her way to a church. I couldn't possibly help Belle tonight. I was the one who needed help. Had God misunderstood my prayer to be rescued?

"I'm sorry, Phil. I can't help you, tonight. I just can't."

He was very gracious and apologized for phoning. The receiver was scarcely back on the hook before God was silently speaking to my heart: *You have just turned down your rescue. I was sending Belle to help you. She is the answer to your prayer. Trust Me.*

I didn't understand, but I dialed Phil back. "Uh . . . Phil, I was wrong. I'll be right over to get Belle. Keep her there. I want her to stay here."

"Listen, you don't have to."

"Yes, I do. God said to. He's up to something."

In Phil's office Belle and I embraced. "Come on, Belle. Supper's ready."

Even as I said it, I realized that all my joy was back, plus some! It was as though the depression had been run over with a bulldozer and squashed dead. I couldn't seem to do enough for Belle. If she'd been the First Lady, I couldn't have felt more honored. She didn't look too great. She was tired and bruised and smelled slightly of alcohol and tobacco. She wore an old hat and layers of clothes against the cold. Her large purse contained empty beer cans.

At my house she wasn't greeted exactly warmly by my children. They had long ago grown weary of my "unusual" friends. Jennifer and the boys silently passed her the food and spoke only if she spoke to them first. If she noticed their coolness, she overlooked it. She seemed to enjoy the meal and had lovely manners. It was obvious that she had come from a family that observed the niceties. Still in pain from physical abuse, she made polite conversation and did not complain. I think her courage was the thing I liked most about Belle. That and her honesty.

"Marion, do you know where there's a prayer meeting tonight? You're always going to prayer meetings." Belle had attended a Bible study one Friday evening here at our house.

"I know of one, but I hadn't planned on going."

"Come on, let's go. Please."

I couldn't tell her no. On the way she started telling me again about how unworthy she was. I'd heard it all before. In the driveway of the home where the Bible study was being held we watched some of the others entering and Belle said, "Oh, Marion, why did I think I could go in looking like this?"

"I know them, Belle, all of them. They've all been through their own private battles with sin and acceptance. They'll receive you with love."

"I can't face them." She was near tears and trembling. "I can't show my face in there."

"Tell you what. We can back in and they won't see our faces."

It worked. Belle threw her head back, laughed and said, "Let's go."

The host met us at the door and gave Belle a big hug. The lesson was about God's unconditional love and Belle cried softly from time to time and held onto my hand until I was certain all the circulation was cut off. As we sang, "Fall down before Him, love and adore Him," Belle gracefully and in slow motion slipped from her chair to her knees and then bowed down to the floor. Alone in the center of the circle she sobbed, "O God, help me. I can't make it anymore. Please do something with my life. I give it to You." In an instant she was surrounded by people loving her, like a swarm of bees hovering over a bent flower. We held her, rocked her back and forth like a baby, brought her tissues, talked to her and prayed with her. When she stood up she was radiant, hardly looking like the same person.

After coffee and cake we drove home. I had planned to let her sleep downstairs on the sofa bed in the recreation room but God reminded me of something. *Remember the night that Jerry had surgery and you hurt so bad you couldn't function? A friend took you home, drew up a bath, gave you a silk gown and a cup of hot tea, and then because you were afraid to sleep alone, she moved her husband into the guest room and let you sleep with her.*

"Hey, Belle, how about a bubble bath? Then you can put some lotion on your bruises." She'd shown them to me, swollen and purple. While I laid out my best gown and robe, I heard her singing in the tub. She came out all scrubbed and shiny, hair brushed soft. We crawled into bed. "Night, Belle."

"Night, Marion."

I was almost asleep when she sat up and said, "Marion, do you think He had a good place to sleep most of the time?"

"Who?"

"Jesus. I mean, He traveled around. I like to think that people were good to Him and gave Him a place to sleep."

Next morning in the kitchen Belle wanted to know how I had peace and joy since Jerry was gone. "Don't you miss him?"

"I could spend twenty hours a day missing him," I said, "but you see, I know he's O.K. and God wants me to be O.K. too. God's taking care of me and knows all my needs. He knew I needed you to come spend the night with me."

She buried her head in her hands. "Not me, Marion. I could never help you."

I took her hands from her face. "I was sinking, Belle, and I asked God to send someone. From all the people that I know, He picked you. I'm very grateful.''

She looked at me a long time, took a breath and said softly, ''You're welcome.'' Then she said, ''But how do you know Jerry is O.K.?''

''Well, from the Scriptures. Believers have certain promises and I base everything I believe on God's Word. And then, I saw with my own eyes. I saw victory and power come into Jerry's life. And in September Julie had a dream and—''

''Oh, tell me about the dream. I have lots of dreams!''

''I don't think all dreams are from God, Belle,'' I said cautiously. ''Sometimes the enemy, Satan, can get into our dreams. And it's so easy to go overboard in interpreting them.''

''I won't do that. Tell me,'' she begged.

Quickly, I prayed, *Lord, she's been so afraid of death for so long. I think You want me to share this with her. Give her understanding.*

''Can I have some coffee? I won't smoke yet. I know you don't like for me to smoke. Just coffee, O.K.?''

''Sure.'' We sat at the kitchen table and I began. ''I had been out of town for two weeks in September. When I got back Julie asked to spend the night here. In the five years she's been married she's only spent two nights at home. The night Jerry went to be with Jesus and the night I came home. I got up early the next morning and came down to the kitchen about five A.M. Julie was sitting over on that tall stool drinking coffee. She had this marvelous, happy expression on her face. I've only seen it a couple of times . . . when she got engaged . . . and when Jamie was born. I knew something special had happened and I hoped she'd tell me. Sometimes Julie is very quiet and ponders things, especially things from God.''

''Did she tell you?'' Belle asked, leaning forward.

''Yes, this is what she said: 'Mama, the most wonderful thing happened last night.' She looked like a little girl again in her pink robe. Somehow I knew not to interrupt or ask questions. She seemed to be caught up in some kind of . . . something. I don't know how to explain it, but I didn't want to break or disturb whatever it was.

" 'Mama, I saw Daddy last night. I talked to him. He was here. Oh, I know it was a dream, but not any ordinary dream. I've somehow been with him, really. It was a gift from God. I'd so wanted to talk to him just once more. I had to . . . and I believed I would.

" 'In my dream or whatever, I was down in the den and there he was. He was sitting in the blue chair. He had on blue jeans and that checked shirt that we like. He had all his hair and he was smiling. He had his tennis shoes on. Oh, he was smiling so big and in the dream he'd already gone . . . you know . . . to be with Jesus. He was here for a visit, sort of. He knew I didn't expect to see him. I ran to him and he opened his arms and held me for the longest time. He seemed to have some new knowledge or something. He looked so wise, like he knew things I could never understand or believe. But it was Daddy, like always. He talked without words. Somehow we just communicated with our thoughts.

" 'Daddy, it's you!'

" 'Yep, it's really me, Julie.'

" 'Did you go to your funeral?'

" 'He laughed. "No, honey, I meant to come, I really did. I heard it was wonderful!"'

" 'Have you seen Jim Tumlin?' (A minister friend of ours who also died of a brain tumor.)

" 'Not yet. He's over in another section. But I can go see him and I will. Julie, I live by a beautiful stream and can go fishing anytime I want to. And tell Mother that it's O.K. Jon's not playing football. I always pushed him too hard about that.'

" 'Do you wish you could come back to us?'

" 'He thought for a moment and smiled at me, the sweetest, most contented smile, like he knew this wonderful secret. "No, Julie. I'm supposed to be here now. This is right. We'll all be together sometime. Things that you think are so important, are not really important. You can't imagine what I've seen here. It's real, all right.''

" 'Mama just got back from a trip.'

" 'That's nice. I'm glad she's not afraid of flying anymore. She's going to be all right, you know.'

" 'Daddy, I'll miss you when you go back. Sometimes I miss you so much and I want to be close to you.'

" 'Come here, Julie. Put your hands in mine.'

" 'I did, Mother, and he had freckles like always and it was his hands—you know how they were square. They were strong and tan.'

" 'Shut your eyes, honey. When you want to be close to me just reach out to Jesus. You know how to do that. You can always talk to Him, can't you?'

" 'Yes, Daddy.'

" 'Then reach out to Jesus just like you're reaching out to me now. You can be close to me by calling on the name of Jesus.'

" 'I opened my eyes. "O.K., Daddy, I'll do that." He hugged me and walked up the steps to the kitchen and started getting smaller and smaller until he vanished, but it was O.K. I wasn't sad. I'd had the conversation that I needed and I got to see him, well—healed! I could tell by his eyes that he was excited to be going back.'

"I listened intently to every word, Belle. I knew it was much more than a dream and also that it would not happen to me. It was some sort of supernatural gift for Julie.''

Belle had forgotten her coffee and sat with her hands holding her chin, listening. "I believe it, Marion. I don't understand it, but I believe it. Heaven is real, all right.''

That afternoon Belle's cigarettes gave out and I'd already told her that I would not get her any more. I had found a program that was willing to take her in, a branch of the David Wilkerson Homes, but she didn't want to go. She began to get restless without the cigarettes and finally said, "I want to call my husband and go back to him.'' I'd been through this before with her and knew no amount of arguing would dissuade her. I took her back to the church where he would come for her, and we hugged goodbye.

That night after I was in bed she phoned. "Marion, guess what? I prayed out loud at supper tonight. A first for me. I asked everybody to hold hands like we did at the Bible study. My husband and the children did it. They looked surprised, but they did it. I know Jesus heard me, Marion. Me! Belle Williams."

An hour later she phoned again, "Marion, guess what? I prayed again. I knelt at the bed and asked my husband to hold my hand and let me pray. He looked funny but said he guessed it was O.K. I talked to Jesus twice today. Maybe it's not too late for me, after all. Keep praying for me, O.K.?"

"O.K., Belle. And . . . thanks, Belle, for rescuing me."

21

The Vacant Seat

This was a wonderful discovery I was making about life on my island: Just as God had supplied all the people Jerry and I needed during his illness, so His representatives continued to appear in my life with uncanny timing. Shortly after Belle's visit I had a chance to attend a large gathering of Christians—probably sixteen thousand or so—in Dallas, Texas. I'd never been to Texas, and when a group of fifteen of us from our area decided to go, the airlines reduced the fare to half price.

Jon and Jeremy weren't overjoyed about my going. I suppose when a child loses one parent, he tends to cling to the other one. I could remember clinging to my mother and constantly being afraid that something might happen to her. I didn't want my boys in such bondage and decided to go as much for their sakes as mine.

At the Dallas Convention Center there was a wonderful feeling of unity and love. In addition to the group of us from home, I bumped into friends from other places whom I hadn't seen in years. Many marvelous things happened during those few days, but perhaps the most enlightening was totally unexpected. Sometimes I wish when God is about to teach me something, He'd hold up a sign and an announcer would say, "May I have your attention, Marion. This is lesson number thirty-six entitled

'Trust,' or 'Patience,' or 'Forgiveness.' " I wish the announcer would add, "Now you won't understand this while you're going through it, but hang in there. You need to learn this. You're ready for this."

The convention was almost over. By now I felt I belonged, not only to my small study group, but to all the thousands present. It was a good feeling. I felt snug and secure.

Suddenly without any warning, as I sat with friends of more than twenty years waiting for the evening meeting to begin, loneliness hit me like a punch in the stomach. Perhaps the emotion was triggered by the fact that everywhere I looked in the vast auditorium were couples. I felt like that little girl of long ago who was uncomfortable with other little girls and their daddies. I wanted to run back to the hotel, but how could I explain it to my friends?

Lord, why are there so many couples? I had forgotten how special it was to be a couple. They touch, pat one another, write notes, share a Coke. Then I noticed that the chair next to me was vacant. That was unusual: the seats near the front usually filled up quickly. *Lord, send someone special to sit there. Someone who'll help me forget about myself.*

The singing began and we stood up. When we sat back down I realized that someone was sitting beside me. I looked at him. He could have been anywhere from sixty-five to seventy-five. He had long, shoulder-length white hair and a white beard. He wore an assortment of mismatched clothes with a large, torn overcoat and white shoes although it was January. The shoes and the coat were too large. Jesus stickers were on the coat and it smelled slightly of mothballs. He was smiling and patting his foot to the music. Contentment could have been his name, or Gratitude.

"Hi," I said.

He turned to me. "Hello." We shook hands.

"My name's Marion."

"Why, hello, Marion, I'm John." As I introduced him to my friends he rose from his chair and bowed, like someone from an old-time movie. Though he had the manners of a prince, he was obviously a street person. Convention members had gone out and invited many people inside.

"Are you a Christian?" I whispered.

"Sure am. Since 1939. Jesus has never failed me and never will, either. Are you one?"

I nodded. As the first speaker stood up I realized that my feelings of despair had evaporated in the warmth of this man's personality. I was glad someone had invited John in and that he'd sat by me. When the meeting was over he turned to me and said, "Well, I certainly enjoyed sitting with you and your friends." I gave him an impromptu hug and attempted to slip a ten dollar bill undetected into his worn pocket. He caught me. "God bless you. Thank you."

I was smiling again on the outside and on the inside. I felt secure and I didn't understand exactly why. I just knew that God was in control and knew what I needed and that He was never going to leave me or forsake me. I knew He sent John to sit with me.

Walking back to our hotel, I asked, "What was that lesson, God?"

I thought I understood Him to say, *Avoid self-pity at all costs. Remember I told you that you could not make it if you indulged in it. It is never from Me. You told Me on May 11th that you would avoid it. Anytime you feel self-pity you are getting off the Island of Trust.*

I got a quick mental picture of myself wading out into the chilly water. Then I got another picture of me hurrying back onto the island and sitting there basking in the warm sun. I breathed a sigh of relief. I guess if God had held up a sign, it would have said: "The faithfulness of God."

Just before I drifted off to sleep the gentle voice suggested: *John belongs in the book you're going to do.*

I made a quick mental note: John—unlikely character. Nevertheless sent by God.

I was actually working on the book now. It was becoming bigger and bigger. It was still only in draft form, but I knew now that it was going to become a book. The first rough draft was written in only seven sittings at the typewriter. It came incredibly fast—often I'd type thirty to fifty pages at a time, not even stopping to think—so different from the way I'd written my other books.

Because the manuscript was getting so heavy I needed something to put it in. I looked through the hall closet and found Jerry's briefcase. I had to smile when I picked it up. Jerry was forever forgetting his briefcase. He'd call home about nine-thirty: "Listen, I forgot my briefcase. Could you meet me at the Gulf station in twenty minutes?"

He couldn't ask me to bring it downtown like most husbands, because I didn't know how to drive downtown. But I could go as far as Medlock Gulf on Ponce de Leon. All the men there knew us. When I drove up, someone would call out, "Hi, Mrs. West. Need any gas, or are you just bringing Jerry's briefcase?"

The case was dark brown and it popped open. I slid the manuscript into it. Then I took it in and out several times because I liked the sound the briefcase made opening. I took it to my desk and lettered across the briefcase with white liquid paper, "Nevertheless." Jon happened by and said, "Mom, you can't paint on a leather briefcase. I can't believe you'd do that."

But I liked it. I traced the letters with one finger. Soon I got into the habit of carrying the briefcase around with me. At night I took it upstairs and put it by my bed. In the morning I brought it downstairs and placed it near my desk. I carried it in my arms like a baby. When I had a few spare moments I'd pull it out and edit, the way many women pull out their knitting.

One Wednesday morning I took the manuscript in the brown briefcase to my prayer group. We were meeting in the 150-year-old log cabin that we used as a prayer chapel. For six years we'd met here weekly. We'd prayed together, laughed together, cried together and talked for hours in that old cabin. It seemed like another home to all of us. Once when I was angry with Jerry at the supper table (he probably wasn't talking to me enough) I ran away to the log cabin and sat there fuming and crying. Soon I heard his car turn in, then the creak of the old front door opening and his methodical-sounding feet. Walking slowly . . . no hurry. We laughed and he held me for a little while. That's all I had wanted anyway. That's why I had ''run away.''

Now I wanted my friends to pray for the manuscript there in the cabin. I held the briefcase in my arms the way I'd been carrying it around the house, like a baby, while the group put their hands on the brown leather. They prayed for each chapter, the cover, the editors, the proofreaders, the printing press, the marketing . . . they prayed for a long time while I held the brown briefcase to my heart.

22

The Restoration Room

The deeper I got into the book, in fact, the more I realized how often, in years gone by, God had tried to bring me into the wonderful dimension of Nevertheless Living—and how constantly I had failed to understand. I'd had hints and foretastes in plenty, all without grasping the principle. Perhaps I simply hadn't been desperate enough. . . .

One evening nine months after Jerry died, Jennifer and I sat in her bedroom making plans for her wedding in the fall. "I wish Daddy could know that I'm engaged," she said wistfully.

"I think he guessed you and Charlie would be married one day, Jen. He liked Charlie so much."

"I wish Daddy could have given me away."

"It's going to be special this way, too." We had decided that Jon and Jeremy would both give her away, walking her down the aisle together.

Jennifer was about to finish college. She still lived at home and worked part-time both for a pediatrician and a vet. Things were good between us now, but it hadn't always been so. She was the child who was the most like me and for a period of time, I wondered if things would ever be right for us. I looked around us, remembering how God had used this room to bring about a healing between us. It had happened two years previously: If I could have learned the secret then, what misery I would have spared myself when Jerry's illness struck.

I don't know when Jennifer's rebellion began. She was so quiet it was hard to spot. I had a two-year old when she was born and then when she was in kindergarten, the twins arrived. They were so demanding and active that Julie—dependable Julie—almost became a little mother to Jennifer.

When Jen was about fourteen I sometimes noticed a sad expression on her face and a tendency to withdraw. Her appetite was poor, but generally she seemed happy enough. I was so busy with the other children, with Jerry and with my writing and speaking that I convinced myself things were O.K. with our second child. I even found time to help other people with their problem teenagers, never dreaming that my own daughter would soon go to others for help. One day a phone call came from a stranger, a young married woman: "I don't know you, but you need to learn to communicate with Jennifer. She is troubled and doesn't know how to talk to you." I was angry and hurt and almost certain that the woman was wrong and I told her so.

By then Jennifer had acquired an assortment of friends that I thoroughly disapproved of. I tried to explain to Jerry why we should break off some of these relationships, but he kept assuring me things would work out. He hated to be firm with Jennifer and I was certain that she needed that . . . from him. "She makes excellent grades," Jerry would insist. "She's O.K." But she was much too thin. At a check-up when she was sixteen, the doctor grimly told me that she was borderline anorexic. "Is there a problem between you two?" he asked. I wanted to scream to him, "I'm a good mother! I've written books and lectured about motherhood."

Jerry continued to think I was making too much of her behavior, her sullen attitude and episodes of disobedience. "It's just a stage," he'd say. In order to compensate for her unhappiness, he began to say yes more and more. He gave her increased freedom and this caused panicky feelings inside me. I felt strongly that she needed more protection and authority—deeper communication with her daddy. Conversations between Jerry and me centered around Jennifer—with me talking 'way too much.

Sometimes Jerry gave Jennifer permission to go places when I'd beg him to say no. She didn't look a bit happier with the granted permission, but she'd glance my way with a look that said: "See, I'm going to get my way. Daddy said so." If she'd actually said that out loud, Jerry could have seen what was happening. But her rebellion was so quiet. And I was so noisy.

Because she wouldn't talk to me, I began to write her little notes, and leave them in her room. I didn't know if she read them or not. But years later I learned she read them until they almost fell apart and carried some of them in her purse at all times.

I became more and more nagging and critical of Jerry. At my insistence we went to seminars and had some counseling. Jennifer's friends called at all hours. I learned to hate the telephone and even to be afraid of it. When it rang a pain shot through my stomach. Sometimes I took it off the hook and once I thought about tearing it out. Jerry told me I was acting like an army sergeant. "Well, somebody has to do something," I snapped back.

Desperately trying to communicate with Jennifer, I asked her if we could pray together one morning before she went to work. She stared at me coldly: "I don't have anything I need to pray about."

I felt like I was hanging onto my influence with her by my fingernails. I suppose that thought triggered my answer. "What about your fingernails? Don't you want them to grow out?"

She immediately shut her hands. "O.K., we'll pray about my fingernails," she said. Maybe she was making fun of me, but we prayed and asked God to help her stop biting her nails. I'd forgotten the prayer when one day she showed me her hands. Her nails were growing! I was so encouraged that I began silently to ask God to restore our relationship. I asked for new Christian friends for Jennifer. I prayed that her daddy could meet some of the needs in her life. I didn't even tell God how. I didn't know. I prayed for Jennifer to gain weight. I asked Him to give her the desire to go to college. She had refused to even talk about going. I asked Him to give her a godly husband when the time was right. Finally, I asked God to help me stop nagging.

There was an eventful night when I asked Jerry while we were eating supper, "Would you consider counseling one more time with someone new? Jennifer has told me that she's thinking about running away and getting an apartment." I saw Jerry grimace at the thought of more counseling. "I have an appointment," I said, "if you and Jennifer will go."

Jerry had chewed his food slowly, thoughtfully. I could have slung mine at him. Why wasn't he answering me? What was there to think about? Right then I heard God's silent voice. *Be quiet, Marion. You talk too much. I am dealing with Jerry. He doesn't move as fast as you do, but he will respond if you will hush.*

I prayed silently, *O Lord, please let him take the authority. Whatever he decides, I'll do. Just let him do what Jennifer needs.*

Jennifer came through the door and passed by us without speaking. "Hi, Jennifer," Jerry said. She ignored him. I clenched my teeth in order to keep quiet.

"Come here, Jen," Jerry called. She came and looked at both of us defiantly. Jerry was still smiling as though we were part of the Brady Bunch. "Jennifer, your mother wants us to go talk with a new counselor and I am in agreement with her. I support your mother. She has a lot of wisdom about some things. You be ready in twenty minutes."

A silent prayer sprang from my heart: *O Father, how wonderful Your ways are! Thank You for helping me keep my mouth shut.*

Jennifer had never openly smart-talked her father before, but tonight her reply was, "I'm not going and you can't make me." Jerry put his fork down and still smiling said, "Jennifer, the three of us are going. We will leave here in twenty minutes. I will carry you to the car and your mother will sit on you while I drive and I'll carry you to the counselor's office if necessary. Is that clear?"

Another prayer sprang forth: *O Lord, did you hear? Why didn't I shut up sooner?*

Jennifer's mouth opened with a surprise at first. But then it tilted slowly upward into a radiant smile. Her eyes danced. I hadn't seen that expression in a long time. She nodded, ran up the steps to change clothes. A long time afterwards Jennifer told me that that evening was a turning point in her life. She said that her daddy was wonderful.

After a time the counselor had Jerry and me leave while he talked to Jennifer alone. When we returned almost two hours later she was crying. He had somehow broken down a wall that no one else had been able to penetrate.

Jennifer had been refusing our hugs and affection. Now she threw herself into her daddy's arms. He picked her up and just held onto her for a long time. I saw tears on his face too. I grabbed both of them and then the counselor hugged us all. We looked like a giant pretzel.

In between sobs, Jennifer said, "Mother, Daddy, I want to ask you to forgive me for the sin of rebellion." She nailed it right on the head. No self-justification. "I forgive you, Jen," Jerry said.

"I forgive you too," I said.

Things were a lot better after that, but somehow I sensed that something else had to happen. Jerry and I were in Sunday school a week or so later when the teacher spoke of forgiveness. "If you have any unforgiveness in your heart toward anyone, you have put that person in bondage. Even if you're praying night and day for that someone, God can't answer your prayer because your unforgiveness stands in His way." I started to cry and people stared, but I didn't care. "Even if you have said that you forgive someone," the teacher went on, "you haven't if your heart still hurts. The only way that person can be set free is through your complete forgiveness. When you have truly forgiven a person, your heart won't hurt anymore."

I was certain God was speaking to me. As soon as we got home I went to Jennifer. "I didn't really forgive you, there in the counselor's office. Not in my heart. I'm sorry. I meant to, and I said the words, but I guess I wasn't ready. I am now, Jennifer. Right this instant, with God's help, as an act of my will, I forgive

you . . . totally. It is as though you never did anything wrong. I
was wrong, too. I need your forgiveness."

She looked at me. A long, searching look. I had almost never
admitted that I was wrong about anything. "O.K., Mama. Sure."
I wanted to hug her, but I knew she wasn't ready right at that
moment, so I didn't. But I believed right then that we would one
day hug spontaneously again. She went to her room and for the
first time in years, my heart didn't hurt.

That was early October, 1981. That Christmas Eve, standing
by the Christmas tree that she had decorated with soap suds for
Jerry, Jennifer told us, "Mama, Daddy, I've been praying about
something. I know I'm not in God's plan for my life. God wants
me to go to college and I want to go. I want to go to Mercer here
in Atlanta and live here at home with you . . . under your authority." It was the most wonderful Christmas present ever.
Shortly after that Jennifer began getting involved with the college
department at church and made lots of new friends. The following March she asked permission to go to Florida with the college
department on a retreat.

After we saw Jennifer off on the bus, back at home for some
reason I walked into her room and sat on her bed. It was a disaster
area. It seemed to symbolize our relationship. Dirty, scarred . . .
in shambles. We'd had so many ugly scenes in that room.
Screaming, threats, tears, accusations . . . tears welled up in my
eyes as I looked at the room and remembered. . . .

Redecorate the room, came the powerful thought. *Restore the
room even as I am restoring your relationship with Jennifer.*

"Sure," I temporized. "I'll make up the bed, vacuum, pick up
her clothes. . . ."

*A complete restoration like the completely new relationship
you and Jennifer are about to have. Get busy!*

I had no idea how to wallpaper and I knew if I asked Jerry to
help me he'd read the instructions for three days. I can't make
sense of instructions and there wasn't much time. When I got
home with the wallpaper I prayed, "In the name of Jesus, wallpaper, you are going up, straight and right." And it went up in

record time. I worked for three days almost non-stop restoring the room. Jerry even cooked supper one night to allow me to keep at it. The finishing touch was a photograph that I searched through the attic for. It was of Jennifer and me when she was four months old. I was holding her and we were looking at each other intently. I put it in a calico frame and set it on the freshly painted antique dresser. Finally, I turned on the new little lamp by her bed and collapsed on the floor. I could hardly remember the bad times; they were gone forever. I'd never been so tired or happy.

I had to be somewhere when Jennifer got in the next morning. As soon as I got home I rushed up to her room. Her bags were stacked neatly in a corner, her beach coat hung up. She hadn't unmade her bed with the new spread and little pillows, even though she'd been sitting up on the bus all night. She'd simply curled up at the foot of the bed like a kitten. She woke up and saw me looking at her. The next instant she was in my arms. We held onto each other for a long time and then sat on the bed and laughed a little and cried a little. "Oh, Mama," she sniffed, "it's the most wonderful room in the whole world and you are the most wonderful mother." Then she said, "Something special happened at camp. I've met someone . . . he goes to our church. You've seen him around . . . you'll be seeing a lot more of him. His name's Charlie."

Now as we talked in that room, planning her wedding, I realized how soon it would be empty. How many lessons this room represented . . . about the relationship between forgiveness and answered prayer . . . about God's power, as He promises in Joel, to restore the years that the locusts have eaten. But the basic lesson, the secret of Nevertheless, had eluded me until later. Things had not changed for Jennifer and me until the night I relinquished my "rightness," my timing, my program—until I heard God say, *Step aside, Marion. You can do nothing. I and only I can do all.*

It had taken a mortal illness to convince me that this was true in every case . . . all the time.

23

The Conversation

Jon and I were becoming close now, too. Once he said, "Mom, we were never close when Daddy was alive. It's sort of fun getting to know you." For my part, I was constantly seeing new things in him that I admired. He never complained, almost never lost him temper. Both his strength and his weakness was his phlegmatic temperament. He wasn't highly motivated, except about a few things—like eating and playing tennis. Like Jerry, he didn't talk much, but he was an example of the old saying, "Still water runs deep."

It was nearly a year since Jerry's death. I had learned by this time that the enemy never gives up: Loneliness and depression would always try sneak attacks on me. But I was learning, too, that somehow God would rescue me. He would intervene if I remained on the Island of Trust.

That June afternoon the tempting voices were especially strong. *You're dreading tonight, aren't you? You're going to be alone, you know. All the children have plans. Could be depressing.*

I stretched out on my bed and stared at the ceiling. Outside the window the lawnmowers being pushed by husbands in the neighborhood hummed. *If Jerry were here, he'd be doing something in the yard, too.*

Our yard looked wonderful. Jeremy had assumed that responsibility and we could have gotten yard-of-the-month, if there'd been such an award. It was a big job, but Jeremy handled it cheerfully and I never had to tell him to cut the grass.

Jon sat down on the bed by me. At one time Jon and Jerry had had such a close relationship that I used to feel almost jealous; they'd talked together forever. Jon was just the age now of Jerry when I first met him, thirty-two years ago, and like his father in so many ways. Like Jerry he had difficulty expressing deep emotions.

Even though we were getting along well in some areas, we'd been arguing about responsibility, his wanting to drive, girls, picking up his clothes, helping Jeremy in the yard . . . the whole bit. His voice had been gruff recently. He thought I was too hard on him. I guess I had a real need to hear him say something good about me.

He stretched out on the bed by me. "You're going to be late for the party," I nagged, just as I used to nag Jerry about time.

"It's O.K.," he laughed. "Nobody wants to be early for a party." His voice was different—gentle, soft. He hugged the pillow on my bed and stared at the ceiling with me as though we were watching television. I recognized his mood. He was that much like Jerry.

"Jon, you have something on your mind. Just say it."

"Naw, Mom. Nothing. Just not ready to take my shower."

"Jon, what is it?"

"Nothing, Mom." His voice was still unbelievably gentle.

Minutes passed. He was struggling with unspoken words. I could almost feel them inside him. "Mom, you want me to stay home tonight?"

His words hit me unexpectedly, like sweet syrup running all over me. I didn't want him to miss the party. I guess I just wanted him to offer to stay. I didn't know I needed to hear those words until he said them.

"Oh, no, Jon. I want you to go."

"You didn't eat supper. Where will you eat?" he asked.

"I'm not hungry. You know food's no big deal with me."

"I could go with you somewhere and talk to you while you eat. I have to eat at the party . . . if I go."

"Thanks, Jon. Really, I'm not hungry tonight."

"I've been thinking about some of the things you said at school." I'd done a little teaching on creative writing at the school he and Jeremy attended. Jon had begged me not to come. "You might say something weird," he'd insisted.

"I'm coming, Jon. I hope you live through it. I want to do this with the students." I hadn't thought he'd listened to me at school. He'd looked at his feet most of the time.

Now Jon said suddenly, "I could probably write an essay about when Daddy died."

I was stunned. The children didn't like for me to write about them most of the time. They didn't think it was so neat for their mother to be a writer. At once the teacher in me took over. "What did you learn from this experience? What was your turning point? Was there an unlikely character who helped you?"

"I guess you were the unlikely character, Mom."

"Me! I didn't think you approved of anything I did. You even said I seemed to have too much joy."

"I know. But now that I think about it, you didn't fall apart or anything. Didn't scream. Didn't even cry. You just smiled and kept on going. You were very efficient with all the plans and all. I like efficiency."

"Jon, I have to tell you something. Before I finally let go of Daddy and decided to trust God as never before, I thought about killing myself. I'd done so many things wrong as a wife. When Daddy got sick, I suddenly learned what was important, and then he was going to be gone, just when I'd gotten it all together. It seemed so totally unfair."

It was perhaps the longest conversation of our lives. Jon hated what I called meaningful conversations, just as Jerry had until those last months. "Mom," Jon asked, "how were you going to kill yourself?" We were both still lying on our backs staring at the ceiling. The late afternoon sun cast shadows in my bedroom and the lawnmowers still hummed.

"I thought about going around that curve on the expressway too fast. You know, the one where the students from Emory do research?"

"But, Mom, there's no cliff there. You just would have gone into the grass. You wouldn't have killed yourself."

I sat up on my elbow. "Really? I thought I would have. It looked like such a good curve. . . ."

Jon started to laugh. Slow at first, then faster, like a train gaining speed. He had Jerry's dry sense of humor. He curled up in a ball, holding onto the pillow and laughing. I laughed, too. "Oh, Mom, you would have messed that up good. Sometimes you really mess up things. Remember the time you cleaned Daddy's paint brush by putting it down in the gas in the lawn mower?"

We laughed until our stomachs hurt. Afterward Jon asked, "What are you going to do when we're all gone?"

"I don't know. It's not my problem. I belong to God. He'll have to figure that one out."

"Would you ever get married again?" The question was totally unexpected, but it was an honest one and deserved an honest answer.

"If that's God's plan for my life. I'd like to love someone again."

Still looking at the ceiling, he said, "I think that would be a good idea, Mom. But you know," he chuckled softly, "it would have to be someone that was . . . a nut like you. I mean, you do weird things. And he'd have to be a real Jesus freak."

I laughed again. "I know, Jon. Just an average somebody wouldn't work. I'll always do weird things and Jesus will always be first, no matter what."

We both kept looking at the ceiling, silently now. "Mom," he said suddenly, "you're crying! You never cry. You didn't even cry at the funeral."

I couldn't explain. They were sweet tears, though; tears of gratitude for the unexpected conversation, Jon's open concern, his genuine love, his humor, his gentleness, his encouragement.

As I finished my victorious cry, he said, "I really don't care about the party. I'll stay home tonight."

Enough tears. I got up. "No. You're going. I'm fine, better than you imagine. Finish getting ready." When he came back to the bedroom, dressed up, I saw him looking at my red-rimmed eyes. "I know, Jon, my eyes don't look right. I'll wear dark glasses driving you to the party."

At his friend's house I let him out. "Have a good time." I drove home alone and went into the house alone.

Nevertheless, I wasn't lonely.

24

Happy, Happy Birthday!

July 8th arrived. My birthday. It was a Sunday. I woke up early and looked out the window. Just as the sun was coming up. I always woke up early now, to look out my bedroom window at the new day. Each day excited me as though I'd never seen a day begin before . . . as though I'd lived most of my life a sightless person. What would God do today? What would He teach me? What could I teach someone else? The days were so different now. I wasn't afraid of sunrises anymore . . . or of the countless decisions and problems that would arise daily like the sun. What a magnificent thing to wake up fear-free!

At a recent Bible study someone had asked how I was doing. I had replied, "Well, I look out my bedroom window each morning, expecting something wonderful. It wouldn't surprise me to see a burning bush or a host of heavenly angels standing in my yard."

"Don't overlook the robin hopping around in your yard," one in the group said. "He's from God, too." This particular morning my yard appeared to be full of robins.

I rested a bit longer, listening to the praise music coming from my favorite radio station. Someone was singing, "Great is thy faithfulness, O God my Father . . . Morning by morning new mercies I see . . . All I have needed thy hand hath provided. . . ."

I propped my elbows on the window sill, recalling Jennifer's birthday, just two days before mine. I'd been looking for paper to wrap her gift in. I found some beautiful pink and blue wrap that I'd liked so much I'd saved it to use again. As I pulled the paper from the drawer, I remembered where it came from. Jerry had wrapped my birthday present in it two years before. Unexpectedly a small white enclosure card fell out and slipped to the floor. I picked it up. There was Jerry's strong, familiar handwriting, the way it looked before he got sick. I read: "Happy, Happy Birthday! I love you. Husband." Funny, I didn't ever remember seeing the card before. Somehow I must have overlooked it: I was seeing it for the first time today.

Happy, Happy Birthday. He'd never used that expression before. The card suddenly became more than a birthday message two years old. It was for now—and it was a wish for a lifetime. Jerry wanted me to be more than just happy.

What's more than just happy? What's beyond happy?

Joy! "I do have joy," I said aloud. I put the small white card on the kitchen table. It was a powerful encouragement and I knew it was from God as surely as if He'd hand-delivered it to me. If the enemy could read I wanted him to see it.

I had asked the Lord to let me do something special for Him on my birthday. As it turned out my Sunday school teacher, Brenda, had called on Wednesday to say she'd be out of town on Sunday and to ask me to teach. Three weeks previously while Brenda had been teaching, I'd had a strong desire to raise my hand and share a little about Nevertheless Living—just a sentence or two. But my hand wouldn't move. *Wait,* God seemed to say.

Now as Brenda spoke on the phone, I thought God said, *Go ahead.* I agreed to teach: I'd celebrate my first birthday after Jerry's homegoing by presenting the Nevertheless Principle to a small group of women. What a birthday present from my Father!

Still lying in bed I remembered that just a few days ago Julie and Ricky, with Jamie and Katie, the new baby, had gotten home from vacationing in Florida. I hadn't seen them in a week. They lived only ten minutes away. I drove over and, since the door was unlocked, let myself in. The house was toy-strewn. A pile of unfolded diapers was in the middle of the floor with Katie laughing and kicking on a blanket beside them. She was ten weeks old now. I recalled how the doctor who had delivered her, a good friend of mine, had motioned me back to the delivery room when she was just a few moments old. He had been Jerry's friend too. A radiant Julie put the baby into my arms. Holding her I remembered Jerry's words just two weeks before he left, when speaking was so difficult. "Julie, God is sending you another baby. You'll see." From that first moment I saw Jerry's expression in her tiny face. It was incredible, she looked so much like him. A few weeks later when she began to smile I noticed that before the smile reached her mouth, there was a hint of it in her dark eyes . . . just the way Jerry had smiled. There in Ricky and Julie's living room I knelt down and bent over her and she gave me a Jerry smile.

"I'm bathing Jamie," Julie called from the bathroom. "Be right out." Jamie preceded her mother, running to me minus her clothes and gave me a big, wet hug. "Hi, Nanny! I went to Florida and I wasn't afraid of the ocean." Julie came in and plopped down on the sofa. "Ricky's at work," she said. "I haven't had a chance to get myself cleaned up yet." How well I remembered those days when there wasn't a minute all day long for myself and the house would never stay picked up. "Tell me about the book," she said. "How far are you? Do you have the ending yet?" She was glowing as only the young, very happy can glow. She didn't even know she was glowing.

"No, but it'll come."

"I bet you'll go to important places now, and do big things. I think I always knew you would . . . someday."

We looked at each other for an unguarded moment with the two children and the mound of diapers between us.

"Julie, there isn't anything any bigger or more important in life than this. My being able to be here with you. This is big time . . . nothing will ever be any bigger in your life or mine than a day like this. . . ."

She smiled a funny little smile and suddenly her brown eyes sparkled with tears. Mine did, too. We both looked down and began folding diapers. We didn't often say deeply emotional things.

Still in bed, that birthday morning, enjoying my thoughts, I let my eyes roam around my bedroom. My mother had given me an antique bed and I'd redone the room around it. Ricky had put in a white ceiling fan. It squeaked and he wanted to take the squeak out, but I thought it was a companionable sound. I'd found an old white trunk and an antique dresser and chest. It was a different room, now, and I was a different person. The old Marion would have been terrified of this solitary birthday. She would not have looked out the window or enjoyed the robins' song. It felt good to be this new person.

My eyes kept moving about the room until they stopped on the birthday present that Jennifer had given me last night. It was a magnificent beige briefcase—my favorite color—with lots of zippers and compartments. Really smart looking. Jennifer had been unable to read this book as I worked on it. Julie had read each word hungrily and made suggestions, but Jennifer had cried uncontrollably the few times she tried. So last night when I'd opened her gift, I was stunned. Jennifer has a knack about color and style. Her room may be a mess, but she's the fashion coordinator for the whole family. Even the boys ask her about clothes.

"I wanted you to have the right kind of case for your manuscript. You'll probably be traveling and I . . . just wanted you to have it. It matches most of your clothes." I took the manuscript from the brown briefcase and placed it immediately in the new one. "I love it," I beamed. Then I noticed there was a letter with it. I suppose it was the letter that I'd longed for all during those long, difficult teenage years that Jennifer and I struggled through.

> July 8, 1984. Happy birthday, Mother. You've always said you'd love to get a letter or poem on your birthday, so this year I decided to do it. Since this is

your last birthday I'll be home, I wanted to make it special.

Mother, I love you. Over the years you have demonstrated genuine love to and for me all my life. It seems just yesterday you were saying, "One day you'll look back and see I'm doing this because I love you." I never thought I would.

But it's so clear now. You loved me enough to risk my acceptance of you and I thank you for it. I have seen the Lord work many miracles in your life and in our lives together as mother and daughter. I praise Him for that. Thank you for encouraging me never to accept less than the Lord had in store for me. I know that if it hadn't been for your listening to the Holy Spirit many times, my life could have taken quite a different direction than it did.

Mother, I know God has many, many wonderful blessings in store for you. He is going to use *The Nevertheless Principle* in a powerful way in many people's lives. I can't wait to get my copy and sit down and read it. I love you very much. Jennifer.

It was only last night that I'd read the letter, and already I had almost memorized it. Its contents were for me like the balm of Gilead.

The sun was fully up now. It was past six. I went downstairs still in my pajamas, as I did each morning, and out the back door. I sat on the back steps and looked out over the yard. It was freshly cut, countless dew drops clinging to blades of grass so green they almost didn't look real. I remembered the Scripture that God had given me along with that list of twenty-six people I needed to forgive. When I finished walking through it with Jesus, God gave me 2 Samuel 23:4:

"And he shall be as the light of the morning, when the sun riseth, even a morning without clouds; as the tender grass springing out of the earth by clear shining after the rain."

A robin ate at the bird feeder. The day was cool and new. Caleb, our collie, came over and put his head in my lap as he does each morning. "Thank You, Father, for this happy, happy birthday. Thank You that I'm not lonely or afraid or anxious about anything. Thank You that I have no fear of the future. Oh, I know there are a lot of things that I could be worried or anxious about. There are things I could be stewing about this very minute. . . .

"Nevertheless, I choose to trust You not only for a happy, happy birthday, but for a happy, happy life."

My joy was rooted so deeply that I thought, *This could well be the most joyful day of my entire life. So far* . . .